A Thinking Proce

MW01078966

by

Dr. Michael J. Hammes

ISBN: 978-1983539527

There's nothing either good or bad but thinking makes it so.

Shakespeare

Introduction

A major challenge in life is to create an effective thinking process that will lead to a healthy mental, emotional and spiritual state of mind. A state of mind that can successfully navigate the ups and downs of life. That is, by effectively processing our feelings, learning new lessons from our experiences, develop effective coping strategies, and to move on with an effective living process. One that will help us experience purpose, meaning, love and hope. We don't live well without these attributes.

Recently, Ms. Cheslie Kryst, a former Miss USA, committed suicide by jumping from her high-rise apartment. She was 30 years old. She was smart, beautiful, outgoing, a charismatic personality, and had opportunities for financial benefits. In essence, she had the good life, which is what most people dream about. Yet, something was wrong with her living process, which added fuel to her inner turmoil that negatively influenced her perception of life. This in turn, influenced her thinking process that led to her committing suicide. What went wrong? Then there is Simone Biles. She had difficulty competing at the Olympics because she was unable to stay focused on her events and decided to not participate in all of her events. She was not in the right state of mind.

Mental and emotional health problems are being experienced by the masses across the country. Looking at the data, most people are not doing very well. Their mental and emotional state of mind deteriorates through the everyday stresses and strains, which causes one's thinking process to malfunction. Overtime, their emotional misery increases, and their solution often about mood altering, which only provides short term relief. A recent headline on the internet, just reported that U.S. drug overdose deaths has increased by 30% during the pandemic. Clearly, more evidence of people getting consumed in their failed living process, not being able to effectively cope with emotional misery, and losing hope. Consequently, their bad thinking process continues to make bad decisions, which only causes more harm to their mental/emotional health. In this case, suicide is the worst decision. Furthermore, over 23 million individuals are addicted to alcohol and drugs (Drugfree.org 2021). This is roughly equal to the population of Texas. Then there are over 300,000 individuals who visit the ER every year for self-harm injures (National Health Statistics, 2018). Also, there were over 47,000 suicides reported in 2018, which includes the over 23,000 suicides by firearms (National Health Statistics, 2018). In case you didn't know it, we live in an addictive society, and by the time most people turn 40, most people likely have an addiction. What went wrong?

Let's think a second about the volume of violence that occurs because of suffering from mental, emotional and spiritual health issues. For instance, every minute, 20 people in the U. S. are physically abused by an intimate partner. This equates to over 10 million men and women in a year (Statistics ncadv.org). In addition, many individuals/families are unable to manage finances, which only increases stress levels. Then, there are millions of children displaying

4

Table of Contents

Additional books:

**A Workbook for Creating an
 Effective Thinking Process: 2ⁿᵈ Edition**

Simple Ways To Create More Available Money

All are sold on Amazon.com

severe behavioral issues, like an eating disorder, drug problems, withdrawal, etc. Let's not forget the homeless and the school dropout, who end up in gangs and eventually, in prison. Do you ever wonder why? Do you have a sibling, or cousin or a life partner, who is an addict, or is living a messed up disordered life? I could go on, but I am sure you get the point. Because of their poor mental and emotional state of mind, they are losing their sense of self, and eventually, get consumed in their dysfunctional living process. What follows are acting out behaviors that help alleviate their inner emotional turmoil. This is only a short-term fix that often becomes a lifelong habit, and or an addiction. Life will never get better. These are symptoms of a living process that reflect mental and emotional health issues that were caused by severe painful emotional issues experienced during childhood, which lead to a flawed self-definition and a flawed thinking process. This in turn leads to making bad decisions with bad outcomes that becomes a troubled living process that lacks meaning, purpose, love, and hope. We don't live well without these attributes. The country pays a steep price for ignoring this problem. The blueprint that creates our failed living process is comprised of the following components.

Flawed Thinking Process

Flawed Self   +   Flawed Emotional   +   Flawed Mindset   =   Bad Decision
Definition   System   Making

The purpose of this text is to describe the development of a failed thinking process that leads to a failed living process. The cornerstone for our failed thinking process is a flawed self-definition that is influenced by raw feelings and emotions, thus, the creation of a distorted realty, and bad decision-making. In addition, a discussion about learning an effective thinking process that will lead to good decision-making, which is guided by logic and reason, related to goals, healthy boundaries, and our well-being. In essence, how to nurture and love our self. This process begins with an admission that our living process is guided by impulsive decision making that leads to a troubled living process. This admission is important because it is about believing one is not a victim, and has the power within to change, and to create a healthy living process.

An Effective Thinking Process

Hlthy Self   +   Effective   +   Effective Mindset   +   Everyday Living   =   Life Outcome
Definition   Emotional   (Options, Tech Skills)   (Psych Needs)   Good Decisions
(integrity)   System   (Rules & Guidelines)   (Goals, Vision)
(dignity)   (Essential EI, Beliefs)

The first task is to examine your living process, and then your definition of happiness and success because most people have the wrong definition. It must include love of self and love of others because life encapsulated with love will be a very meaningful life. This sets the direction for your life! Then work from left to right beginning with addressing past unresolved emotional core issues, which allows the real you to come into being. Then learning how to create an effective emotional system and an effective mindset. This will set in motion the development of an effective thinking process that empowers one to make good decisions based upon self-love, healthy boundaries, logic and reason. It also will allow your consciousness to expand, which will lead to a greater good and illumination. This becomes the spiritual journey.

Chapter 1: The Journey

Happiness is what everyone wants, but few ever experience it. To begin with, happiness must be defined, so we know what it is. Happiness is an experience that is dependent upon the following things: 1) peace of mind, 2) experiencing harmony, 3) finding your passion, 4) coping and managing well with the highs and lows, 5) having love in your living experience, 6) creating and enjoying a simple life, 7) being centered and balanced, 8) able to nurture yourself, 9) being adaptable, and 10) being resilient. More items could be added, but these seem to be most essential, and spell out that happiness is much more than a smile or sleeping late. Also, peace of mind and inner harmony are the prerequisites for experiencing happiness. Few people ever experience happiness, and it is not fun to wake up every day and have a depressed outlook on the day and for the future. Consequently, many people live in a state of depression and anger, have a loss of meaning, purpose, love, and hope, which becomes a life never lived. It is not a surprise that people mood alter to ease their misery that comes with not being happy.

To experience happiness, we must also understand the concept of mental, emotional, and spiritual health. Think of these as a computer program that can help us experience peace of mind, harmony, and happiness. Let us begin with mental health. Mental health includes our emotional, psychological, and social well-being. It affects how we think, feel, and act. It, also helps determine how we manage stress, relate to others, and make choices. Mental health is important at every stage of life (Mental Health.gov. 2020). We must understand how good mental health is imperative for creating and living a healthy living process. A living process guided by an effective thinking process that enables one's ability to manage the everyday living process, and significant life changing events.

Life is a journey but has become a messy difficult troubled journey because of our poor mental and emotional health, which leads to our flawed thinking process. Because we chase the good life, our journey becomes a very emotional stress filled experience that will challenge our meaning, purpose, hope, and love. We do not live well without these attributes. Sustaining these attributes, especially hope, is dependent upon our ability to develop and grow with our difficulties, and not lose hope. Losing hope means we have surrendered to our disordered painful living process because we are not able to create solutions. We struggle when we lose hope because hope provides a lift in our spirit and provides the incentive to keep fighting through our challenges to create new meaning and purpose. Presently, hope for many is fragile because they lose their sense of power because of their inability to successfully manage their emotional struggles, which often becomes overbearing. The usual outcome is getting stuck in one's own self-doubt, self-pity, and negative feelings, and emotions, which usually lead to confusion. Many get lost amongst their confusion and chaotic living process, and just live with their emotional misery, which becomes exhausting. Consequently, many people live day to day, and rely on mood altering experiences for feeling alive because this is what they have learned to do, and it provides a temporary relief from our madness. Yet, this leads to a troubled living process absent of growth, and the spiritual aspect will wither away.

Think of a flower that is growing in your yard. You fail to nurture the root system, and the flower blossoms, but dies early. However, if you would have nurtured the root system, the flower would be much stronger, more resilient, have a brilliant shine when it blossoms, and shine for a longer period. Most people live a similar living process because they fail to nurture their inner sense of self because they lack self-love and live with a flawed thinking process that erodes our sense of self. We just do not know how to nurture our self and lose our sense of self in the struggle of everyday living.

This flawed thinking process leads to bad decision-making and bad life outcomes, which leads to a troubled journey. It is a decision-making process misguided by powerful feelings and emotions that have come from painful childhood experiences that have been repressed in our unconscious. Often, we do not even recall these painful feelings and emotions, but they are alive and well within our unconscious, and interfere with our thinking process for the rest of our life. Sadly, our thinking process becomes an automatic process governed by these buried feelings and emotions, and by our raw feeling and emotions that are created by painful living experiences. Consequently, we just do not know how to think differently, but we do the best we can, yet we still end up with a miserable living process. Recently, reported as a news item, the suicide rate for men in their fifties, has increased by 50%, which strongly suggest that there is something wrong with their living process. Specifically, as it relates to their lack of self-love, purpose, meaning, and losing hope.

An effective thinking process must be able to effectively process information through our foundational beliefs. This is difficult but is necessary to create an accurate reality. We make decisions according to our reality, which must be accurate, or we make bad decisions that lead to bad outcomes. In addition, our thinking process must be guided by self-love because this provides the foundation for creating an effective thinking process that can create purpose, meaning, hope, and love throughout our lifetime.

An effective thinking process will also help navigate one through the intense difficult periods of significant loss, and the change that follows life changing events. Such events will challenge our belief system, and our experiences of meaning, purpose, love, and hope. That is, if our thinking process does not process our feelings and emotions in an efficient healthy manner. Most people will often allow the event to define them in a negative manner. Then we see ourselves as a victim, which takes our power, and then become vulnerable to bad decision-making. That is, we will engage in destructive coping behaviors that only makes the living process worse for all involved, or we will just give up, and go through the motions of living.

The overall result will be a diminished sense of purpose, meaning, hope and love, which often leads one into a state of depression and anger. If not processed, our negative state of mind will totally suffocate the human spirit. Our life becomes an empty experience because we live and experience life through our anger, which paralyzes our thinking and there can be no joy. However, often our life changing events, regardless of how painful, and can be a serendipitous moment because it may function as a wake-up call to examine our belief system, our values and priorities, and how these influence our meaning, purpose, love, and hope. In addition, to examine our thinking process and decision-making process. This introspection is how our consciousness grows and expands, and with this comes wisdom that has always been within us. We just needed a push for it to come to the surface and be a part of our thinking process.

Our flawed thinking process has been partly programmed that the wonderful life and happiness that we chase is guaranteed. That is, if we get educated, get a good job, make good money, get married, have children, and have money to buy many toys. Many people do all of these things, or some of these things, and then one day wake up and realize life sucks. Our kids are acting out, you or your spouse is having an affair, or has a drug problem, maybe a family member is experiencing anxiety attacks, or has an eating disorder, etc. You ask: Why me? How can this be?

Think of this as working hard to get to the top of the ladder, and one day you get to the top, but then realize the ladder is against the wrong wall. Now you are left with an empty feeling and do not know what to do about this. This is the image of the good life that most people chase, but lose their sense of self, and most of what the important things are in life, along the way. This often leads to a mid-life crisis. Asking the above questions is the first step in realizing your living process is failing and a change is needed. Admission that your living process is failing is the second step. There can be no growth without admission. Furthermore, it is important to accept responsibility for your failed living process because your bad decision-making created it. Also, realize that you are not a victim, and you can change your living process.

The following are questions that can help stimulate a new journey.
* Have you realized the life you have isn't the one you want?
* Have you realized that happiness will not be experienced regardless of how hard you work and how much money you make?
* Have you ignored your physical health and are experiencing health problems?
* Are you drinking too much, not spending enough time with your loved ones, have you had affairs, do you keep attracting dysfunctional partners and don't know why?
* Do you feel that your significant relationship has lost its passion, and you have become roommates?
* Do you live in an emotional prison?
* Do you feel like you are screaming inside and can't be heard?
* Do you feel like you have lost your freedom and power, and feel trapped?
* Are you experiencing episodes of depression and anxiety attacks? Do you wonder why?

The big question is: Are you loving you? Life is really about love, which begins with learning to love you. Has love the price you have paid for chasing the good life?

At some time in life, we get to a point where we need to redefine success. Success must also include efforts for loving and nurturing oneself, creating and maintaining loving relationships, and developing a sense of self-responsibility. Self-love is most important because love is the most important aspect of our living experience. Love provides a base from which to experience joy, purpose, meaning, and hope, which provides direction and a vision. Think about the last time you bought something that was important. For a week or two the item was especially important, but then the item became less important. Things only provide short term value, whereas love and loving relationships last a lifetime, at least they should.

The key ingredient for experiencing love as a top priority is that we must be able to love our self. Then one has a healthy self-definition, which becomes the cornerstone for creating and experiencing a healthy loving relationship. Consequently, one will realize they have a choice in who they love. That is, they have a sense of power, and are not a victim, and are capable to love. Presently, most people are hesitant to get to close intimately because they often view this as a weakness and afraid of losing control. Sadly, such an individual lives with their ego as the control center, which is guided by raw feelings and emotions, fears, and immediate satisfaction. It provides an effective way to live in denial and to avoid their inner painful feelings and emotions. This often leads to problems related to control issues, and or lack of control.
Do you know people with large egos? The result is bad decision-making that leads to bad outcomes and a troubled living process. A very good friend of mine never let anyone get close to him because he was protecting himself. He did not want to reveal who he really was on the inside. He was a very quick thinker and was always two thoughts ahead of anyone talking to him, and he used this to control the conversation, so no one could get close to him. I believe his motor within was running at 10,000 mph, when it should have been at a 100 mph. His emotional system was flawed, and his feelings and emotions were stored in a huge reservoir within, which, I believed caused his cancer. He died before he was 60. Consequently, the consequences of a troubled living process often lead to health problems. This raises the following questions:

* **Are you happy with your living process?**
* **Are you satisfied/happy with your loving relationships?**
* **What kind of living process do you want to experience five years from now?**

The clock is ticking, and we do run out of time, so don't waste time. Furthermore, if you live long enough, you will end up in a nursing home, and your kids may select the one you go to. If you do not end up there, then you will probably die sooner than later, but the question is still the same.

How do you want to experience life between now and then?

How are you doing? Look in the mirror and ask: am I happy? What kind of living process have I created? How do I explain my behavior? At some point in time in the living process of most people, they one day realize the life they are living is not the one they want. At this point, it is important to realize that you are not a victim and can learn to create a new healthier living process. In addition, one can begin the process of unlearning the way they have been taught to live and learn a new way to live. This is difficult because it requires a new and unique way to think, but we do not know how to completely change our thinking. Furthermore, changing our thinking process becomes more difficult with age. Assuming you are somewhat of a balanced individual and have some mental capacity to view your life objectively. I think you will agree

that no individual wants any of the following experiences. Are you experiencing any of the following?

1. No one wants to spend any part of their life in jail or prison?
2. No one wants to get into a troubled relationship?
3. No one wants to be hurt by someone else or to hurt someone else?
4. No one wants others to manipulate or exploit you?
5. No one wants to give their freedom to someone else?
6. No one wants their friends to make bad choices for you?
7. No one wants to live a life of extreme loneliness?
8. No one wants to be dependent upon others for your happiness?
9. No one wants to be poor?
10. No one wants to experience a life that is full of misery and pain?
11. No one wants to become an addict?
12. No one wants to become mentally or emotionally disabled?
13. No one wants to die young because of a bad decision?

The failed living process of today, is the modern-day disease. It is caused by a flawed thinking process that is created during early childhood. At the base of this flawed thinking process are unresolved core emotional issues that have been repressed into our unconscious. Consequently, this buried emotional matter will manifest into a damaged mental and emotional state of mind. The result is a flawed self-definition that becomes the cornerstone for the development of a flawed thinking process. Consequently, many people lack healthy boundaries, which causes our thinking process to malfunction. Furthermore, the flawed thinking process often becomes guided by raw impulsive feelings and emotions. This in turn leads to a distorted reality that creates a lot of confusion, which a flawed thinking process cannot sort out. The outcome is bad decision-making and bad outcomes. Eventually, we lose our sense of self, and our ability to nurture and love our self, and life becomes a troubled living process. Life becomes a difficult journey.

Chapter 2: The Dysfunctional/Unhealthy Lifestyle

If you were in an airplane looking down, you would see the image of happiness because most people seem to be enjoying the many wonderful amenities of our modern society. That nice house, nice cars/trucks, HD TV, boats, and the many other toys that are used for enjoyment. Yes, the good life. However, look beneath this image, and you will see signs of a troubled living process experienced by many millions of people.

* An insatiable appetite for drugs.
* Alarming rates of crime and violence.
* Alarming rates of suicide and suicide attempts.
* Alarming rate of failed marriages/relationships.
* Alarming rate of addictive behaviors.
* Alarming rate of sexual transmitted diseases.
* Kids acting out through destructive behaviors.
* The prevalence of white collar crime.
* Alarming rate of eating disorders.
* Excessive shopping and gambling.
* Don't forget an obsession with sports and sex.
* Extreme hypocrisy from politicians and religious leaders.
* Discrimination.

Look a little deeper, and you will notice disturbing psychological symptoms of a troubled living process, such as: anxiety attacks, nervous breakdowns, frequent periods of depression, periods of severe depression, life dissatisfaction, excessive anger, rage, frustration, and hopelessness. All items listed above are psychological symptoms of a living process gone wrong. Other symptoms include poor time management. Some people work long hours, ignore their families, loved ones, and often ignore their health. Often, the most successful people are also very dysfunctional in their personal lives, and in their interpersonal relationships. Then others do the least amount of work required, and just survive because they are lazy, which carries over to other areas of their life, which never leads to a good outcome. Usually, this imbalance of time commitment and energy is often for the love of money, self-validation, and or being lazy. These symptoms are related to a lack of self-discipline and misplaced priorities that cause many other stressful problems that produce more emotional misery for them and their loved ones.

Another symptom is when the main priority for many people is to make money and a lot of it, which is how we are programmed. This is about misplaced priorities that creates serious life problems. Many people become consumed by this desire, and often sacrifice their most important relationships, which is a steep price to pay. One may have great wealth and a lavish lifestyle, but symptoms of misplaced priorities are displayed when a family child develops an eating disorder, or engages in drug use, drops out of school, and maybe attempt suicide, and the parents wonder why.

Furthermore, many people also have a spending problem, and need more and more money to pay the bills. This problem overrides the most important priorities of loving relationships, and consequently, their living process will begin to unravel. In relation to these issues, is that the more things people acquire, the more pressure there is to make more money because as a rule most people are never satisfied and want more. However, this chase for more money and things, increases the emotional stress and strain on the everyday living process, which eventually, overwhelms the individual, and or family.

The solution to their money mismanagement was to make more money when all they had to do was underspend, learn to be satisfied with less, and then they would have enough money. In addition, they would not have all the emotional stress. Money is nice, but it cannot buy purpose, meaning, love, and hope. This is the price most people pay in their chase for what they think is the good life.

Some people believe a troubled living process is a result of bad luck. He/she is drinking because of a bad life experience, or what most might label as bad luck. There is good luck and bad luck. In some instances, there is bad luck where one can just be in the wrong place at the wrong time. However, in many instances we create our own bad luck. Examine bad events and determine the process of how you arrived in that situation, and you will see that you probably created the bad luck by making bad decisions that was guided by powerful emotional impulses. Furthermore, anyone who has a troubled living process is always stressed because they are always doing things for the wrong reason, which leads to making bad decisions that creates crisis after crisis. They might see this as bad luck, but it is bad luck they have created caused by bad decision-making often based on emotional impulses. For instance, it is common for people, when under a lot of stress, to regress back to old unhealthy habits that provided pain relief. However, these unhealthy habits always lead to more bad life outcomes. In essence, they keep repeating the same mistakes repeatedly, which is often viewed as bad luck. Discontinuing bad decision-making is extremely difficult because it is what they have learned to do. On the other hand, people can also create good luck by having an effective thinking process guided by healthy boundaries that lead to good decisions and good luck will be outcome.

Evidence provides a very clear picture that we are not prepared to create a healthy living process in our modern society. Consequently, many begin to experience more frustration, anger, anxiety, and depression. These are life killers because they suck life from us, and we have less energy to nurture ourselves and for our loving relationships. Sadly, there is no solution in sight because of living with a flawed thinking process. At some point, the individual becomes mentally, emotionally, and spiritually bankrupt. To escape this misery, many people rely on a quick fix to ease their misery. Alcohol, cocaine, meth, sex, eating, and spending money, are the most common choices used to create a quick fix. Eventually, for many, these unhealthy habits become addictions, which take control of the thinking process, and life gets progressively worse. Sadly, everything else in their living process becomes less important, including significant loving relationships. Eventually, the life of many individuals goes up in flames because their life begins to unravel, and then becomes a complicated mess that produces more misery and less hope, with no solution in sight.

One thing for certain, a troubled living process will create an empty disordered life, which becomes complicated, messy, and painful. Eventually, the living process spins out of control, destroy lives, and loving relationships. Look at: John Edwards, Mel Gibson, Arnold Schwarzenegger, Charlie Sheen, Bill Clinton, Mickey Mantel, Marilyn Monroe, Jim and Tammy Bakker, Michael Jackson, O.J. Simpson, Steve McNair, Lindsey Lohan, Elvis, Amy Winehouse, Harvey Weinstein, Matt Lauer, and Charlie Rose. Don't forget Tiger Woods and Bill Gates.

All of these individuals had it all, that is, fame and fortune. What they had was not enough, and they had to self-medicate because love is what they could not do. Their flawed thinking process failed them. People who love themselves do not throw away their life by making bad decisions, but admit they have a problem when the symptoms appear and seek professional help.

Dysfunction in the Workplace
Not long ago, a disgruntled employee in Orlando, Florida, who was fired, returned, and killed five employees, and then killed himself. Today, worksite violence, and gun violence, has become a common weekly experience, which reflects extreme societal and community dysfunction. There appears to be a lot of people who are living on the edge, are pushed over the edge, and then there is a complete malfunction of their thinking process because they lose all rational thinking. Obviously, most people do not kill others, however, there are many people whose lives are unraveling because they lose their way within the stressors of their troubled living process. Consequently, their sense of self becomes diminished along with their meaning, purpose, love, and hope. These are substituted with anger, which is a short step away from violence, and often, more and more people quickly resort to violence. The above is but one example, however, other symptoms include: worker burnout, dissatisfaction by salary and wage issues, harassment issues, fear related to bullying issues that are added to the individual's personal issues, and discrimination. Add these together, and you get low productivity and the potential for worksite violence. These are all related to issues of mental and emotional health issues that can quickly tip an individual to violence. The ill-effects and high cost of stress within governmental agencies, the corporate world, and within the educational system have come to the forefront but should not be surprising.

Unmanaged, emotional misery negatively impacts performance, innovative thinking and the monetary cost is in the billions in the corporate world. The effects of too much stress include fear, anxiety, anger, frustration, suicide, and burnout. These will lead to a negative attitude that affects job performance. The results of this can be seen in the serious problems and consequences at GM. Process evaluation would have identified the ignition problem and saved millions, but someone dropped the ball, and looked the other way. Sadly, at least 13 people have allegedly died because of their failed ignition problem, which reflects corporate dysfunction. Recently, the news also reported the severe consequences of job stress in Japan. The pressure to succeed has become extreme, which has significantly increased the suicide rate for employees. Unfortunately, the flawed thinking process of the corporation, and of the individual, could not solve the problem of extreme stress, and suicide is a very steep price to pay, which could have been prevented.

Most employees in a bad work environment, eventually, cope by mood altering, skipping work, work less, and find ways to get even with poor administrators. Some reach a breaking point, and retaliate with violence, and some commit suicide. Generally, miserable employees struggle to manage their time, which impacts productivity. Other sources of stress come from being mistreated by peers, from inadequate administrative policies, and the stress from a poor worksite. It is not an accident there are increased episodes of worksite violence, and if not appropriately addressed, will only become more frequent.

School Environment
Public education is constantly under a microscope and is blamed for many problems, such as, school dropout, gang involvement, crime, and drug related issues, and not effectively preparing students for the workforce. In addition, in the last decade, school violence has become a new serious societal problem. Recently, a middle school student in Albuquerque shot, and killed another student, who was being the big bully. Some of these problems might have been prevented if schools would deal with emotional issues of troubled students. The problem begins when a child grows up in a toxic family environment and develops an unhealthy mental and emotional state of mind. However, schools can address these issues by changing the educational framework. Presently, society views the student entering the system with an empty head, and after twelve years of being on the assembly line, their head will be full of knowledge that will lead to becoming a functioning citizen. This is true to some degree, but today the system must do more than just provide knowledge. In addition to learning math, science, and English, the educational experience must also prepare the student to be successful in managing their living process that includes learning to create healthy boundaries, to value loving relationships, to learn how to nurture oneself, to learn to ask for help when in need, learn to manage money, and learn how to manage feelings and emotions. In essence, to learn how to better manage their living process by learning to make better decisions that ensures their health, and their future.

Updating the system must begin with the creation of a new educational framework that addresses the entire issue of not learning, and or not wanting to learn. The focus for the dysfunctional student has become the need for self-validation and acting out begins, which puts the importance of learning as being least important. To add to this problem, schools fail to provide help when students demonstrate symptoms such as giving up, performing poorly, and acting out in class. The core issue for these behaviors are emotional issues related to a poor self-definition that needs to be addressed. A new old problem that has come to the forefront is bullying behavior. This is most harmful for the bully and the victim, and both need professional help to address this behavior, and for the harm it causes to the victim. Bulling behavior has a negative impact on learning behavior because students are not equipped to effectively manage extreme emotional distress of fear, anxiety, and insecurity. They feel vulnerable and unprotected, which is understandable. They also fear that if they seek help, they will be seen as being weak, which only creates more fear and anxiety. Unchecked, this dysfunction will continue well into their adult/professional career. In addition, this dysfunction will carry over to the workforce, and not to mention, the emotional devastation within the inner circle of loved ones. Presently, prisons are full of young people that created a troubled life because of their unresolved emotional issues that led to a flawed self-definition, and a flawed thinking process.

This is an unhealthy state of mind that negates the value of education, destroys their future, the value of living a healthy life, and becoming a productive member of society. In their short life, their unresolved issues often manifest into the criminal life that could have been prevented. Efforts aimed at emotional issues can prevent behavioral problems in the future. Perhaps, one day, society will realize the benefits of addressing unresolved emotional issues during the educational experience. Such a strategy would be much easier, and financially cheaper, than waiting till the individual ends up in prison. Such educational assistance can go a long way in healing emotional issues. In addition, to empowering the student by creating an effective thinking process that leads to good decision-making that leads to good outcomes.

Corporate Environment
Innovation begins with imagination and has been the basis for everything that has been created. A creative thought that becomes a concept is usually fostered by a safe environment that stimulates a creative thinking process. The corporation that creates such an environment will often become the leader in innovation, which leads to good earnings. An unhealthy work environment in the corporate environment creates fear, frustration, anxiety, and anger. This toxic environment hinders creativity, basic job performance, and corporate earnings. The underpinning of this problem is a flawed thinking process of the managers that creates a culture of fear and complacency. Today, the best corporations create a safe work environment, and recognize the needs and issues of the employee, in addition to providing monetary fairness. Such an environment will enhance the imagination and creativity, which is required for success.

Corporations that have an unhealthy work environment, usually, have managers and administrators that often use their power for their advantage, and not for the big picture of the company. Look at the Volks Wagon Corporation and see the mess they are currently experiencing. The misuse of power is like being a bully who uses his/her power for their gain at the expense of other employees and the corporation. This practice is a means to acquire the perception of more power, control, and a feeling of importance, which at times is experienced as a short term high. The bully will harass the person they perceive is most vulnerable and use verbal and body language to intimidate them. The individual being bullied will often experience fear, uncertainty, and anxiety, which adds up to stress, and a lot of it. Eventually, the victim of bullying will not want to come to work and will not enjoy their work. Without intervention, good employees may begin to look for different jobs, or file a lawsuit against the corporation for not taking corrective action. In essence, bullying behavior and other destructive practices, create an unhealthy work environment caused by a flawed thinking process that inhibits creative thought, innovation, and negatively impacts corporate earnings.

Community Dysfunction
We all grew up in a dysfunctional home of some degree and have emotional scars to show it, but we also grew up in a dysfunctional community. In large cities, dysfunction makes the news, but in small towns it is the local gossip, such as, who is having an affair, or how much money someone lost at the casino, or who lost a job, or who is getting divorce, etc. Also, there are neighbors who dislike each other, who compete against each other, and neighbors who do not talk to each other. Every community has their alcoholics, the workaholics, the gambling addicts, abusers, etc., and we all interact with these individuals. The accumulative effect of the community is a collective dysfunctional consciousness, which has a negative influence on our thinking process and our development.

Furthermore, we have learned defense mechanisms that helped us survive within our dysfunctional communities, which we often carry with us when we leave the community. Besides the obvious dysfunction, most everyone grows up in a culture of drinking alcohol, and therefore, everyone drinks because it is what people have learned do, and it serves well as a mood modifier. There are many functioning alcoholics that do not even know they are an alcoholic. Another present-day example are tattoos. Another is wearing jeans with holes up and down the front part of the legs. Then there are young males that wear their pants with the belt buckle so low, they have trouble walking. Let us hope they never have to run because their pants will fall off. Yet, another is when the individual stretches their ear lobe, then cuts a hole in it, then inserts a ring into the hole.

Why would young people do these things? They lack a healthy self-definition, and these behaviors are an effort to create a superficial identity. Besides, everyone else is doing it, and is a way to feel accepted, and or just to be different. However, allowing others to define you is a problem because the focus is on a superficial identity, while your true sense of self is ignored.

More specifically, the individual's identity is often sacrificed, which will lead to a flawed self-definition, a flawed thinking process, and bad decision-making. Overtime, an individual will often lose their own potential sense of self because they will get lost within their feelings and behaviors related to their superficial identity/self. Sadly, the life they experience is usually on the wrong road characterized by a day-to-day mentality of making decisions based upon raw emotional impulses related to a false identity. Unfortunately, most young people do not ever consider the short-or long-term consequences of their decisions. Consequences are ignored because their feelings for attention, and their need to belong, override logic and reason, related to their long-term goals and health. For example, someone who has a drinking problem is symptomatic of not learning how to nurture their true sense of self, and there is a disturbance within their inner sense of self, and then lack wholeness.

Another part of our dysfunctional community is that perfect family, in which everything appears normal, and all is well. However, behind this vail of perfection are issues of power and fear that rule the family, which are issues of control. This extreme control often creates an environment of extreme fear, which creates a toxic environment. Consequently, family members are hesitant to express feelings and emotions for fear of being punished physically and psychologically. This gives birth to the development of a flawed self-definition, which will rule their lives and lead to a flawed thinking process and bad decision-making. The healthy development of their true potential will never happen. Evident, is that we not only experience dysfunction in our immediate family, but we get a double whammy by the influence of the dysfunctional community norms and destructive behaviors. This makes it difficult for a young child to think beyond the community norms and to create a different healthy living process.

The Good Life and Suicide: The Breaking Point
A few years ago, I received word that a friend had committed suicide. Of course, everyone in the community was in shock and could not understand why this happened. Jim was married, had children, a lot of money, and all the wonderful things money could buy. They had the good life, at least by the norms and standards of society. Jim was very smart, had a lot of common sense, good looking, had a great work ethic, and all the attributes required for success in the business world. However, he was a failure at the interpersonal level and the personal level. Looking back, there was a deep reservoir of anger within him, which is common in addicts. Everyone near him could feel these vibes of anger and kept their distance because they feared that the wrong gesture of some sort might turn his anger to violence.

Jim grew up in a very toxic family environment, which was characterized by a lot of emotional turmoil because his parents had to deal with their own emotional issues and addictions. Consequently, the mood and atmosphere of the family environment was very unstable and unpredictable, which is a very toxic environment for the healthy development of a child's sense of self.

Unfortunately, his parents were emotionally unavailable for Jim and his siblings. This led to the festering of deep inner core wounds to the human psychic, which are known as unresolved emotional issues, which gave birth to his flawed self-definition and flawed thinking process. His life was characterized by anger, power/control issues, and trust and love issues that dominated his living process. To numb his misery and failings, he developed a reliance on alcohol, which became an obvious addiction during his twenties. It was during this time, his marriage began to fail, and his dependency on alcohol became more powerful because other parts of his life became chaotic. What little love he had in his life was quickly fading. His living process became an empty chaotic experience with little meaning, purpose, hope, and love, despite the monetary success. The accumulative emotional pain was getting progressively worse, which increased his reliance on alcohol. Alcohol became his best friend because it provided pain relief for his misery and helped him make sense of his living experience.

When an individual becomes an addict, they do not realize the depth and power of their addictive behavior because of denial, which allows them to see what they want to see and not what is (Nakken, 1996). Denial is a defense mechanism generated by a flawed thinking process that protects their addiction. Addictions are about having ashamed-based identity that manifest as a flawed self-definition that leads to a flawed thinking process. If you love yourself, you have a healthy self-definition and will not make bad decisions that cause self-inflicted misery. Furthermore, you will be able to create healthy boundaries, effectively manage feelings and emotions, and make good decisions. Jim was unable to do any of these tasks because of his denial and living with a flawed thinking process. Alcohol was his way of running from his painful feelings of himself and his painful emotional issues. With time, he became increasingly isolated because his relationship with his wife grew progressively worse. Eventually, the need to escape his troubled living process grew stronger and stronger, and the power of addiction took total control of his thinking process. His drinking deteriorated because his life spiraled out of control. This is the usual outcome when life becomes an extreme disordered troubled mess, and meaning, purpose, love, and hope have diminished. At this point, it is common for a sense of panic to become part of the thinking process because life is quickly unraveling. In essence, the addict is losing control when control is what they must have.

Near the end, his wife informed him that she was leaving the marriage, and the combination of this failure, and his intense internal pain became too much to bear. His flawed thinking process prevented him from effectively managing the situation and took him to a very deep level of depression and anger, which paralyzed his thinking process. His suicide was triggered by the accumulative effect of his emotional misery, and the moment his wife left him. His dysfunctional life was put in motion when his parents created a toxic family environment, which was absent of adequate love that led to his flawed self-definition. The result was the development of a flawed thinking process, bad decision-making, and a failed living process. His life became a toxic experience, and the only solution was to cope by creating a relationship with alcohol. Eventually, he reached a breaking point mentally, emotionally, and spiritually, and never even considered to reach out for any kind of help. His addiction and troubled living process could have been treated, if he would have recognized, and admitted he had a problem, and then participated in therapy. He did the best he could but was doomed to fail because of his flawed thinking process. Sadly, his siblings also became alcoholics. Sadly, he was not the only causality in the community, as there were two other suicides in the community, before the end of the year.

This is one example, but there are many similar examples in every community when a flawed thinking process of a dysfunctional individual progresses to the level of being out of control. The most notable are the shootings that have happened at Sandy Hook, Las Vegas, and Florida. The shooter reached a point of total collapse for any form of rational thinking. Such a situation reveals the level and severity of the many individuals who have lost their sense of self, and have become mentally, emotionally, and spiritually deranged. They just could not implement a coping strategy for their emotional misery, and never learned that all they had to do was to reach out for help. Subsequently, their confusion and anger, took them to, and over the edge of insanity. The reactionary solution became violence. A thinking process out of control that developed from a lack of love.

Summary
Despite having the many wonderful amenities provided by modern technology, we are not a very healthy happy society. Quite amazing when you stop and think about this for a few moments. Most people have little restraint and are guided by their ego, live moment to moment, and lack the ability to effectively manage their feelings and emotions. This comes from a flawed thinking process that creates a distorted reality, which is defined by confusion, and seeing what one wants to see. The result is reactionary thinking controlled by impulsive needs, wants, and desires, and anger. This usually leads to doing whatever it takes to feel good because this is what matters. The outcome is a troubled living process. Over time, many people become addicted to their coping behaviors, which then controls their thinking process. Life then becomes centered on their addictions, and loving relationships will be compromised, as will their sense of self. Eventually, they will become mentally, emotionally, and spiritually bankrupt, which leads to an empty living process, and the suffocation of the human spirit. This is the journey that leads to the demise of purpose, meaning, hope, and love, and is not the journey you want.

The good news, is that a troubled living process can be changed. One can learn a more effective thinking process, which will help in making better decisions and create a better living process. The most effective way to deal with a troubled living process is to first admit there is a problem, then seek professional help that can heal unresolved emotional core issues and learn a new and effective thinking process. The accumulative affect is the creation of an effective thinking process that leads to a healthy living process. **What kind of life do you want?**

A Flawed Thinking Process: The Beginning
Scot Peck (1979), a psychiatrist, discovered that every one of his patients had an undeveloped spirituality, or a very immature spirituality. Consequently, their life was dysfunctional, or more

specifically, they were living a troubled living process characterized by bad decision-making that led to bad outcomes. In essence, they experienced little or no meaning, purpose, love and hope. These are the attributes that nurture our growth, development, the human spirit, and enrich our life. Without these attributes, the human spirit suffocates. Consequently, the spirit of an individual withers away. Peck also believed that dysfunctional individuals lacked wholeness, which is a disharmony between the personal conscious mind, and the personal unconscious part of our mind (Peck, 1979). The result is a dysfunctional living process characterized by a flawed thinking process and a dysfunctional living process.

Our mind is comprised of three parts: the personal conscious, personal unconscious, and the collective unconscious (shapeinmind.com/2020/02/04/carl-gustav-jung). This disordered relationship between the personal conscious mind and the personal unconscious, leads to a flawed self-definition, which becomes the cornerstone for the development of a flawed thinking process. The personal conscious mind houses the ego, which has access to accessible knowledge, thoughts and experiences, and our accessible feelings and emotions that create our self-definition, and our reality. This includes our belief system, our sense of self, and our filters that shape our reality. The ego commands our thinking process, which is often stimulated by emotional impulses, and without healthy boundaries, often leads to bad outcomes. Our conscious mind is created from our experiences, all our knowledge, our imagination, the amount of anger we have within, our religious indoctrination, our belief system, our family environment, our self-definition, and our unconscious and the collective unconscious. Collectively, the interaction of these components and variables, whether life experiences are pleasant or painful, are summarized, which the mind stores in its mental library. Accumulatively, the information within our library creates our consciousness, which produces our reality. Seems simple yet living has become difficult because the reality for most people is a confusing reality, which leads to bad decision making and bad outcomes. The question becomes: why?

Then there is the unconscious part of the mind, which interacts with our conscious mind. The personal unconscious contains wisdom, and is God, and is also a place where we repress our painful memories and feelings, created from painful events. These repressed feelings were once conscious, but when repressed are not readily available to the personal conscious mind. The reasons why we ignore the unconscious is because we look for God outside of ourselves, and we just do not know how to tap into this important dimension. Most people look up believing God is up above us when all we must do is to look within ourselves. Consequently, we disconnect with God, and this disordered relationship gives birth to a diminished consciousness, and our evolving spirituality, and the human spirit. In addition, most people fail to effectively manage their painful feelings, and repress them into the unconscious, which only makes the already existing disordered relationship worse. Furthermore, the repressing of painful feelings into the unconscious, makes it exceedingly difficult for an individual to connect with the unconscious. It creates a barrier and prevents an individual from making the unknown from becoming known. Effectively managing feelings can take one to a deeper level within their unconscious. This in turn often leads to the enhancement of our sense of self, and our consciousness. More specifically, a healthy alignment between the conscious and the unconscious, creates a sense of harmony and inner peace. In addition, one becomes aligned with God. However, this alignment with God cannot happen when we are looking for God outside of our self, ignoring our unconscious, and/or when we are ego driven and guided by our emotional impulses that are an attempt to please our immediate wants and desires. The outcome will be a troubled living process.

Then there is the collective unconscious mind, which is an internal cultural experience between people made up of images and thoughts, which have universal meaning and are passed on to all generations. For instance, many people fear being in the dark. That is, people experience fear when the lights go off, and the house is in darkness. Then, they hear a noise in the basement, and the combination of being in the dark and hearing a noise, becomes quite scary. This fear of the dark is a universal experience. Most people on the planet also fear snakes and will not even go near a snake. The concept of God is a concept we all share with the entire world. Religions all point to a higher power, which originates from our personal collective unconscious (shapeinmind.com/2020/02/04/carl-gustav-jung). Our thinking process is an interaction of these three components of our brain. Unfortunately, very few people know little about the function of these three components. Consequently, this gives way to a flawed thinking process.

A flawed thinking process does not effectively process information accurately when our reality is distorted. Reasons why include the mentioned variables above, however, being stimulated by emotional impulses, not effectively managing stress, our ego, and having a quick temper, all will short circuit any thinking process. This often leads to a flawed reality. Furthermore, we all have some repressed feelings from painful childhood experiences, however core trauma events cause the most damage. Individuals, who have experienced core trauma events, often repress the associated painful feelings and emotions into the personal unconscious. This is our emotional garbage bin where we discard our painful feelings when we are unable to effectively process them. It is a quite common practice because we do not do well with extreme painful feelings. Sometimes, an individual will bury painful feelings so deep that the individual fails to remember them, and the event that caused them. However, we fail to realize that just because we no longer remember these painful feelings when we repress them in the unconscious, does not mean they are not active.

There are times, when our repressed painful feelings are quickly activated and rise to the surface when new painful experiences happen. This might happen when an individual quickly becomes short tempered, violent, and or communicates with an extremely elevated voice. It is the ugly side of the individual, and often leads to violent behaviors. Furthermore, repressed painful feelings silently influence our conscious thinking process, and often lead to making bad decisions with bad outcomes. For example, an individual may unconsciously fear commitment because their parents were never available for them during childhood. Consequently, this individual is unable to commit to a loving relationship because of their fear of abandonment. This is the unconscious silently messing with our conscious thinking process. Another example is when a control freak marries an individual with no power or control. In other words, this individual has a very flawed self-definition, and in this individual's mind, he/she never measures up to anyone else. They look in the mirror and he/she see themselves as an inadequate individual. Such an individual could be in a room with three people, or a 100 people, and see themselves as the most inadequate individual in the room. The control freak married this individual because unconsciously, he/she knew that they would have all the power in the relationship, and that their partner would be dependent upon them. Thus, he/she would never leave them. Unfortunately, we think we are in control of our thinking, but our unconscious, unknowingly silently takes over our conscious thinking process.

Presently, the living process experienced by most people is created by a flawed thinking with a flawed self-definition as the cornerstone. Because we lack wholeness, we experience insecurities, which interferes with our thinking, as does our impulsive feelings and emotions. In addition, to what is repressed within our unconscious. The result is a disordered relationship between the conscious and the unconscious. As a result, our flawed thinking process creates a distorted reality that reflects our feelings and emotions. Unfortunately, we make decisions according to our reality, and often our reality is a very confused reality, which will lead to bad decision-making. Look at the substantial number of people who believe the covet virus is a hoax, and refuse to get vaccinated, and to take precautionary measures for preventing the spread of infection. Sadly, the death rate is much higher than it should be for people not getting vaccinated. Unfortunately, people are making this decision with their flawed thinking process, which is controlled by their ego. Their paying a steep price for seeing what they want to see.

We also experience frustration and anger when we run into people with a different reality than ours. We may have to change our reality, change theirs, or give into their reality, or live with the one we have, and disconnect from those who think differently. This is what we do, and we try to make sense out of this reality that we have created, but it is difficult because it is a confusing reality. This is exactly what is going on in the country at this very moment. The thinking of the extreme right is controlled by their unhealthy ego, which is influenced by their repressed anger that has risen to the surface and has taken control of their thinking process. That is, they see what they want to see, and not what is, which leads to an angry response, like the insurrection on Jan. 6th. Presently, their inability to negotiate creates a very scary problem for our democracy.

Furthermore, we often experience frustration and stress when life does not satisfy our expectations, which shapes our reality. Many people experience extreme stress when a life event forces a complete meaningful change of life. That is, every aspect of one's life is turned upside down, in the sense that all meaning, purpose, love and hope, will have to be recreated.

This period in an individual's life becomes overwhelming in the sense, the individual will struggle, just to get through the day. To adjust to the new living process, a change in consciousness is required. Without a significant change in consciousness, the individual will have to live in continuous emotional misery, and there will be no joy. When you change your perception, the thing you are looking at will also change, and this is much easier than trying to change the thing you are looking at. We run into trouble when our thinking process lacks the ability to be flexible, tolerant with the existing reality, and the reality of others. When we lack this ability, we then see what we want to see and become consumed by our emotional misery. In human terms, eventually, we become mentally, emotionally, and spiritually exhausted, when we see what we want to see. In essence, we are lying to our self, and our life becomes a big lie. We live with significant frustration, depression, and anger, which is usually repressed within. Furthermore, these repressed emotions, our anger, and feelings, will paralyze the thinking process. This is the price we pay when we do not have an evolving consciousness that leads to an accurate reality.

This disordered relationship between the conscious and the unconscious was created when we experienced our childhood in a dysfunctional family that was rich in emotional turmoil. In essence, there was an absence of nurturing loving behavior, which was substituted with a deadly experience of confusion, chaos, and fear, within the family, which was internalized and create a flawed self-definition, a flawed thinking process, and bad decision-making. A flawed thinking process is also created when one is brainwashed with a specific religious doctrine. In both cases there will be a disharmony between the conscious and the unconscious, which in time, leads to the suffocation of the human spirit. This disorder begins in infancy because an infant lacks a sense of self, and it is during the first year that they develop a sense of self from unconditional love. The parents accomplish this by holding the child, cuddling it, talking to it, singing to it, and praising it, with a degree of predictability, which creates a sense of security. These behaviors are statements that sends the message that the child is special, worthy, and valued, which forms a healthy self-definition. This is a core belief for a child that will become the cornerstone for experiencing a sense of confidence, an inner sense of security, and a sense of wholeness, and harmony.

When a parent(s) does not create an environment of continuous love, the child will develop a flawed sense of self that will manifest as a deep feeling of being flawed and defective. Consequently, this feeling becomes a self-portrait that reflects their perception of self, which is a flawed self-definition. This then sets in motion the development of a flawed thinking process, which will lead to bad decision-making that just does not work well regarding a healthy development. Furthermore, parents are not able to provide adequate messages of love when they have addictions because their addictive behavior is more important than the child. Also, when parents are needy because they must take care of their needs first, and everyone else is last in line. In addition, if parents suffer from depression, and or mental health issues, and if there are traumatic life changing events within the family.

Parents can also provide confusing messages when they frequently say, "I love you", and then turn around and verbally abuse, and or physically abuse the child. The child will then have issues with trust and love. Events as divorce, when a child is in their formative years, will have a harmful effect on the child's development of a self-definition, as will a long military deployment, and a death of a parent. These events are about traumatic loss and change that lead to chaos and confusion that will lead to core emotional issues. Consequently, to a disordered relationship between the conscious and the unconscious that lead to a flawed self-definition and a flawed thinking process. A child must have a strong sense of security and predictability during their first two years of life. This will create the cornerstone for the development of a healthy self-definition.

Furthermore, childhood is not an easy time. Children are very needy and require a great deal of attention from parents. However, in a dysfunctional family, parents are often dealing with their own issues, and the stress related to raising family. Like most parents, they fail to give enough nurturing attention to the child. Consequently, a child will create a defective mindset and an emotional system that will mismanage painful feelings, which helps them survive the family dysfunction. The overall outcome is living with a flawed thinking process that can only create a troubled living process because of bad decision-making. Purpose, meaning, love and hope are pushed to the side, and we just do not live well without these attributes.

In essence, we all, too some degree have some unresolved emotional issues from growing up in a dysfunctional family that lead to some degree of a flawed self-definition. The process of emotional issues begins because a child lacks the ability to effectively manage their painful feelings when believing no one loves them, and or when they feel flawed and defective. The only recourse they have is to repress their painful feelings, thus, the birth of a flawed emotional system, which becomes the operating system for managing feeling and emotions. Sadly, most people use this system for the rest of their life, which robs them from opportunities to grow and become the person they were meant to become.

Yes, bad decision-making, sometimes is about people doing crazy abnormal things, which can cross into the arena of mental illness. Mental illness and being dysfunctional are usually about a self-definition that is extremely flawed and defective that leads to a flawed thinking process. This in turn, creates an alarming, distorted reality, which is often guided by impulsive feelings and emotions, especially anger. In addition, it is also about a mental, emotional, and spiritual state of mind that is underdeveloped and characterized by confusion and chaos. Decisions that fail to nurture the health of the individual, will suffocate the human spirit, and create a disordered relationship between our conscious and our unconscious. Thus, we experience a dysfunctional living process void of purpose, meaning, love, and hope.

The unconscious is accessible to everyone, but only if one takes time to listen to our feelings and emotions and dare to go within our inner conscious being. However, most people do not know about the unconscious, about their inner emotional issues, and the significant role these impact our living experience. Consequently, most people just live, and experience life on the surface, based upon their raw impulsive feelings and emotions to feel good, and often, do whatever it takes to feel good. Furthermore, most people do not do well with misery and want a quick fix to medicate their pain. This self-medication closes the door to our inner sense of self and the unconscious.

Consequently, one is then left with a flawed thinking process controlled by impulsive thinking that guides one through the living process, which never works well. The next time you experience a situation that is painful, take some time to process the experience. Perhaps to your bedroom and lying down, you light a candle, listen to nice soft music, and shut down your thinking, and let your mind quiet down. Maybe it is taking a walk every day, having a conversation with yourself, and with the universe. These methods will help you process your feelings and emotions and will take you within your inner sense of self. This process will help clarify your day, create a sense of peace, and connect with the unconscious.

A lifelong task is to develop harmony between the personal conscious and the personal unconscious. The process of discovering what is in the unconscious, and to make it conscious, is a particularly important step in developing a healthy mental and emotional state. That is, the more we make known of the repressed thoughts and feelings in our personal unconscious, the more our personal consciousness is enhanced. Thus, the greater the harmony between our personal conscious and our personal unconscious. In other words, we get closer to the concept of wholeness, which also leads to harmony and peace of mind. In addition, there will be less stress and turmoil in our thinking process, and in the bad consequences of our thinking.

Spirituality
Spirituality is a very important variable for experiencing a healthy life. Spirituality brings the mental and the emotional aspects together within our sense of self, with nature, and the mystery of it all. This bringing together provides a synergistic process for creating meaning, purpose, harmony, hope, and love. As discussed by Peck (1979), people will experience little spirituality in their living process when there is a disordered relationship between the conscious and the unconscious. Consequently, most people are focused on satisfying immediate needs, wants, and desires, while they ignore their self-definition, and the larger picture of our being. Furthermore, most people have a total disconnect with nature. Most people live in large cities, have no, or little interaction, or connection with nature. The closest thing to experiencing nature is going to a zoo, which has an extremely limited connection with nature. We must realize that we are all part of nature, we have an extraordinarily strong connection to nature, and to separate nature from the living process is a mistake. Keep in mind that we need nature, but nature does not need us, therefore, we must have laws to protect nature.
Consequently, a troubled living process will either lack spirituality, or attempt to acquire spirituality through religion. Religious concepts taken literally fail to connect with our

psychological sense of self, and the unconscious because people get stuck in the concepts instead of transcending the concepts. For the most part, religions have taught us that god is up above us and or outside of us. Consequently, we are continually ignoring our inner sense of self, and the god within, which is the unconscious. Furthermore, there are many different gods in the world, and the extremist in every culture believes their god is the only god, and some are willing to die for their god. For thousands of years, every war, then, and today, have been, and is a holy war. Both sides are fighting for their god and believing God is on their side, and that there is some reward in the hereafter.

Furthermore, the goal of many religions is to convince their members to believe that they have all the answers about God and how God works. The fact is, we do not even know all the questions. In addition, there are many gods because everyone tweaks the image of god for their convenience because they see what they want to see. Others blindly accept the god of their religion because this is easy and convenient because thinking is not required. This is also experienced when people get consumed and lost in a cult. In both situations, individuals lose their sense of self and power, which causes significant suffering. Furthermore, please understand that a priest, minister, rabbi, or any religious leader, is no closer to God than you or I. They have all been educated to serve in a functional role, which requires them to dress accordingly, and their actions and behaviors are to reflect the rituals and beliefs of their religion. However, this functional role has not worked well within the Catholic Church because the child abuse issue is anything but godly and has been going on for centuries. Only recently, has the church been forced out of its lies, and has begun to address this genuine issue, but a lot of lives have been destroyed. The leaders of the church believe and were hoping that an abused child will grow up and get over the experience of being abused. The only result was a lost soul!

What they do not understand, is that feelings are real, they matter, and they do not go away. The abuse experience shatters the integrity of the child's sense of self, which creates powerful shameful feelings of self. Furthermore, the child was often told, that if they tell anyone they would be punished by God, which created additional feelings of fear and shame. Sometimes, we bury painful feelings so deep within our unconscious, that we do not even remember them, or the event that caused them. Yet, these buried feelings are deep within the unconscious, and scar our sense of self, and quietly influence our decision-making in a negative way. Not to mention our ability to trust. Consequently, we end up with psychological scars, which will manifest as a flawed self-definition. This scarring of our sense of self creates an imbalance between our conscious and the unconscious, which is also experienced as disharmony within our psychological inner sense of self. Long term effects will manifest as issues of trust, love, anxiety, and confidence, are the most notable. Keep in mind the impact this has on our immune system. Without professional help, the abused individual will experience a very troubled living process because their flawed sense of self will lead to a flawed thinking process that leads to troubled living process.

Furthermore, some religions are about controlling church members by using fear, shame, and guilt, which allows the religion and church to gain control of its members. This control is often about acquiring power and wealth. Just watch the so-called religious leaders that appear on their Sunday programs. They are all very rich, they play on their member's ignorance, fear, and guilt, as their sermons are coded with a touch of hope. They do this under the mask of God to get money, and a lot of it, and they enjoy the power, and their lavish lifestyle. There are also religions that implement rigid rules that determine the living process for its members, which provides the perception of control for the ruling party. Presently, we have been in a very long war with people who live by such rigid rules and beliefs and are willing to die for their god.

The result of many religions is a very structured reality, with little room for the imagination, and the result is total suffocation of the human spirit. In many instances, it is quite common for individuals to turn to their god during times of distress with anger because their god allowed a painful unexpected event to happen. Unfortunately, they feel that God has forgot them, and or God did not reply to their request/prayers. The only outcome is more anger and depression that can last a lifetime. Spirituality can be accomplished through religion, if one can transcend the concepts and recognize the metaphors. However, most people lack this ability and get stuck on the concepts, which smoothers the human spirit. Furthermore, many people will have a flawed mindset, which only adds confusion in their reality, especially when life changing events happen. Consequently, this will also create an underdeveloped spirituality, or an immature spirituality, which leads to a troubled living process.

Spirituality is about expanding one's consciousness and thinking beyond religious concepts. It has to with the mystery beyond the physical reality, as it relates to the interplay of nature, recognizing a higher power, the universe, life, death, and the pain and suffering of life. Part of this mystery is that there are some things never to be known and are to remain a mystery. However, this thinking goes against the extremists and religions that believe they have all the answers. There are religious leaders who believe that they know all there is to be known, which is very arrogant because no one knows all there is to be known.

Furthermore, one must have the courage to challenge their existing beliefs, and to ask new questions that pertain to the mystery of self, life, living, and the hereafter. This examination process, along with our life experiences will provide an understanding of some parts of the mystery, but this process is a lifelong challenge. Spirituality also includes aspects of higher consciousness, self-efficacy, self-actualization, self-love, and self-assertiveness. It is a higher level of functioning, which is dependent upon an effective thinking process that allows one to question and examine their sense of self in relation to the mystery of it all.

Not everyone develops these qualities of higher consciousness or evolves to a higher level of consciousness because they get stuck in their troubled living process and just try and get through the day. In addition, their flawed thinking process has been programmed with religious concepts, many fear change, and many others eventually give up, and accept the religious concepts provided by their religion. This is always the easiest way and most convenient. Change

in a living process and a thinking process is often feared and requires a lot of work and time. To completely change, one must give up on an old way of thinking before creating a new/different way of thinking. This giving up with an old way of thinking will leave a void filled with confusion, which can lead to a sense of living without a sense of purpose, meaning, hope, and direction. Therefore, many people hang on to their way of thinking because it provides some meaning, purpose, and comfort. Maybe they have a comfortable miserable life, but it is predictable, and it is what they know.

The development of one's consciousness and spiritual aspects are usually enhanced when one experience's a life changing event if one gets through the anger. Some people will grow/change more in six months following a life changing event, than most people will grow in their entire life. This is stated in the song Amazing Grace.
Amazing Grace, how sweet the sound;
That saved a wretch like me,
I once was lost but now I am found,
Was blind, but now I see. (Wikipedia)

With this change of consciousness comes wisdom that helps one to see a much larger reality, and more clarity for understanding the dynamics of being human within the life experience. The reality is that everything we need to know is within us, and we need to tap into this reservoir of knowledge, that collectively becomes wisdom, which will enhance our consciousness. This only happens if we ask questions about why we feel this way, then process our feelings and emotions, instead of repressing them.

However, anger is the most powerful emotion one will feel when an unexpected life changing event happens. Significant others can feel this anger and will avoid you because it often leads to bad outcomes, which can lead to a troubled living process. However, individuals who come from a very dysfunctional childhood have a deep reservoir of anger deep within their unconscious. This stored anger can become activated when an unexpected event occurs that produces frustration and anger. For some individual's, this anger takes over the existing ineffective thinking process of the individual and becomes evil. Evil is a very destructive characteristic, which is not normal by any means of the imagination. Thinking enveloped by evil will often attempt to inflict as much pain and destruction possible on another individual(s), just because they want to, and enjoy doing so. Evil people have evil thoughts that are about destroying life, love, and loving relationships.

The evil may manifest as a very nasty tone of voice used in an argument to inflict intimidation, which is a sense of trying to get more power, so they can overtake the other individual. This intimidation can make the other individual feel unworthy and feel ashamed, which is the goal. If you feel that you have this reservoir of evil within, seek professional therapy. History is full of dictators and kings using evil to destroy people. Read the history of Joseph Stalin, who killed approximately forty million of his own people. Of course, there is Hitler, who tried to rule all of

Europe, and historian's state that more than seventy million died in world war II. Presently, Putin is getting ready to invade Ukraine, and does not care how many people die. Allowing anger and evil to control our thinking is like living in a sense of darkness because our decision-making is not about love and nurturing, but rather about getting even, or attempting to control life and destroy others.

Anger and evil become the enemy and paralyzes the thinking process. This is especially true when one is unable to come to terms with a life changing event. Why does this happen? The life changing an event that upsets our belief system and reality because we are unable to make sense of the event. The result is a collapse of our reality, which leads to total confusion in our living process. This leads to a loss of purpose, meaning, hope, and love, which creates an unstable mental state of mind, which is susceptible to bad decision-making. Do you know anyone who got married on the rebound? Think of your belief system as a completed puzzle that describes your living process. It is like a puzzle that takes a lot of time and effort to put all the pieces together. Once completed you trip and fall into the table, and the puzzle falls off the table into many pieces. Now you must put it all back together again. The same thing happens to our belief system when we experience a life changing event, which results in significant confusion about our reality. Furthermore, change requires a lot of time and effort to put the pieces back together. However, unlike the puzzle, the pieces don't all fit, and new pieces have to be created, which is the hard part and takes time.

The reason all the parts don't fit is because the intense emotional pain from the life changing event forces the individual to ask questions about life, to examine beliefs, and to question the why's and how's of living. The first thing many people ask is: why me? The second is to state that: "this isn't fair." These questions will force an expansion of the inner sense of self and their consciousness, but only if one takes time to contemplate the feelings. Think of when you returned to your high school reunion, and you could not help but notice how some classmates have grown consciously and spiritually, and some have not. It is like if the both of you are experiencing two different worlds, and you are, which is why it may be difficult to connect with them. Personal growth and wisdom are limited, or seldom happens, if one never faces new challenges and experiences, or if one becomes imprisoned with anger. One's spiritual growth and potential is related to the degree of difficulties, challenges, and how one manages related feelings and emotions. Creating new pieces for the puzzle of life takes a lot of time, and the emotional work is painful. However, when you create a new piece that fits, you have a new belief system, an expanded consciousness, a new reality, and an enhanced spirituality. Life gets better because your self-awareness is enhanced, as is your consciousness on your spiritual journey.

Hidden Tools: The Brain, Being Smart and having Wisdom, Premonition, Serendipitous, and Intuition and Common Sense.

Life, today, has become overly complicated. Up unto the mid-seventies, family and community structure provided the rules and roles, for how to live, which made life simple. However, these no longer exist. Consequently, people must figure out how to live a life guided by healthy values. Values that create healthy boundaries that guide the thinking making process and decision-making process. Most people have a failed living process guided by a flawed thinking process guided by whatever feels good for the moment, they lack a healthy sense of self, and do not know what is real or what is not real. This confusion creates a troubled living process, in which many people lose their sense of self in all the confusion created by one's flawed thinking process. Sadly, life becomes a disordered mess, which only gets worse in time, which takes a heavy toll on one's mental and emotional health. I am sure you may have teachers, relatives, and or friends in the community that stand above everyone else. That is, there is a sense that they have it together, and they seem to relate to a larger picture. We notice these individuals they have unique features that most people lack. How do we acquire these wonderful features? Let's begin with understanding our brain.

Our **brain** is a wonderful, amazing thing. There is a lot that we do not know about the brain, but we know it is comprised of the personal conscious, the personal unconscious, and the collective unconscious (Shapeinmind.com 2020/02/04). At least, this is what we think we know. The personal conscious is what we experience daily. It contains our ego, which has access to our thoughts, memories, awareness, and feelings. It is the command center for the body, and processes information that creates our reality. The personal unconscious contains all our memories, including buried repressed painful thoughts and feelings that were once conscious. The collective unconscious is, wisdom we have inherited from our ancestors that help us function (Shapeinmind.com 2020/02/04).

Every day we make thousands of decisions, and most are quite simple decisions, in which our brain is in **auto pilot** and automatically runs the process for making decisions without our assistance. It alerts our immune system when a foreign object enters the body and must be attacked. Have you ever driven to a destination, you arrived, and you realize you do not remember much about the drive? I have, and it is a strange experience. I believe that during the drive, I was totally absorbed in thinking about something else. Yet, my brain went to auto pilot, was operating in the background, and made decisions without me being consciously involved in the operating process. I arrived at my destination, got out of the car, and came back to reality. It was like I got lost in time, yet the brain functioned appropriately. Another example is walking down a flight of stairs, while you are having a conversation with someone. You are focused on the conversation and have little focus on how each foot is doing, while you descend the stairs. Your brain does all the calculating for each foot, on each step, so the foot goes where it is supposed to go.

I am sure everyone has experienced the following. You are going through your day in a normal fashion, and you, suddenly think about a friend that you have not seen, nor heard from for many months, or even years. Then, in a few days, you get a call from your friend. How does this happen? Did our thoughts connect with our friend?

Another example, is forgetting to do something that you had planned to do. I am sure you have, early in the day, sat down, and wrote out checks for paying bills. You put them into an envelope, sealed the envelopes, and put a stamp on each. Then you put the envelopes on the kitchen counter, so you would not forget them, when you intended to leave the house. The time comes for you to leave, and you walk right by the envelopes, and forget to pick them up. You get to the car, and a thought happens, you forgot the envelopes. You go back in the house to get them and mail them. Your brain recalled a forgotten thought about mailing the bills and bought it back into your consciousness. Quite amazing. The brain does have the ability to engage in multiple thinking processes at once, without our command. The brain seems to automatically protect us when we are not totally focused on what we are doing, like driving. The brain also can alert us when we forget something. Plus, our mind expands our consciousness with experiences, which is why we see the world differently when we are forty, as compared to when we were twenty.

Collectively, the three components of the brain work together to assist in the development of our self-definition, emotional system, and in our mindset. The interaction of these three components, create a reality from which we make decisions that creates our living experience. Furthermore, we rely on our functioning brain to help us get through the day, to manage the ups and downs of living, and to make sense of our existence. A flawed thinking process occurs when there is a disordered relationship between the conscious (our reality), and the unconscious. The unconscious contains our hidden repressed feelings and emotions, which shadows the conscious mind, which influences our thinking process in a negative way, which leads to bad outcomes.

Now think of your mind as a **storage** unit containing a billion little rooms, in which the brain stores information. Information from all our experiences including our educational experiences, and all other life experiences. Have you ever had an experience when a light bulb goes on in your brain? Then you say: now I get it. For an example, let us say you have been studying the field of investing, and over the years you have read a lot of information about financial planning. Your brain has put all that information in these little rooms. Then one day, you have an additional thought or thoughts, about investing stimulated by an investment speaker, or an article you have just read. Suddenly, the brain gathered all the information out of those little rooms, put it in one room, and even organized it for you, and then the light bulb goes on: I get it.

Another example is golf, which is a very difficult game, and requires several specific muscular actions to be performed well, in order to hit the ball well. When you were young, you had time to learn the correct mechanics, and were surprisingly good at it, but then you got a job, and had to give it up. After years have gone by, you decide to go back to the game. At first, you are quite rusty, but after some practice, you again become that good golfer. The brain, which stored the golf information, recalled it, and you were able to create an old new swing.

Our brain is amazing in that it does many things at once, with the purpose of helping us function well mentally. This in turn helps us manage the day and to process all our experiences. However, our flawed self-definition and our inability to effectively manage our painful feelings, is what comes back to haunt our thinking process. This becomes the main variable in creating the disordered relationship between the conscious and the unconscious. Perhaps, the brain also includes the following features: **premonition, serendipitous, intuition, common sense, and wisdom.**

There is a thing called a **premonition**. It is a feeling, without any evidence, that something bad or good is about to happen, and then the event happens. How could this be possible? I did experience a premonition during the summer of 1979. I was in a large city going to graduate school during the summer. I was pondering the idea of continuing my educational career to obtain a graduate degree, but I did not want to borrow a large amount of money to complete my degree. Then, I had a thought that took me back home to working during my undergraduate experience. Why not go back home, and work at the construction company for about six weeks. I could make enough money to get me through the first year, and then get instate tuition, which would be much cheaper. I put together the plan. One day at breakfast, I was discussing this plan with a friend, and said: I am somewhat afraid to go back and work because I might get into an accident and get seriously injured. Once I said this, I blew it off. Why would I say such a thing?

I then implemented the plan. I flew home and went back to work for a construction company. Two weeks later, I chain flew off a machine and went through my left arm. It almost severed the arm above my wrist. I was alone on a road, out in the country, bleeding very badly, and knew that time was short because I may pass out from loss of blood. I remained calm, and soon arrived at two choices. One was to get into the pickup and go for help, but I did not know how far I could drive. Plus, there was a lot of equipment I had used that was hanging out of the truck, and a machine was connected to the truck, which would make the truck difficult to drive. Second choice was to run to a nearby house and ask for help. The potential problem was that no one might be home, and then it might be too late to get back to the truck and implement the first choice. Still calm, I heard a thought/voice in my mind: do not worry you are not going to die. It struck me because my thinking was about the two options before me. Right at that moment, a truck pulls up next to me and the driver said: get in. I jump in, and they took me to a fire department, and the first responders rushed me to a hospital. Soon, I was in surgery, but I was not put completely under because I had breakfast shortly before the accident, which can cause complications when coming back to full consciousness. During surgery, three times the physician ask for permission to amputate the hand. I said no. Well, that was over forty years ago. My arm is a little shorter and crooked, but it still works. From the accident, I received a weekly compensation that paid the bills and made the educational experience financially manageable. Looking back, it was a premonition, a miracle, and a **serendipitous** event, all rolled into one. If this event would not have happened, my life would have been a very different, probably in a negative way.

Our brain also has a tool known as **intuition**. It helps in the decision-making process. Intuition is believing that something is true based on what one feels to be true without conscious reasoning. I have always been intuitive, and it has helped me make good decisions throughout my life. When I was 12 years old, I vividly remember leaning against the kitchen wall at home and felt that something was wrong with a certain member of the extended family. However, I quickly disposed the thought because what could I know at 12 years of age. Well, 28 years later, I discovered my intuition was correct because something did happen to this family member, which really, unknowingly, impacted many other family members. Intuition also served me well in making personal decisions such as: going on to school, relationships and marriage, retirement, financial planning, and looking at the future. In every situation, there appears to be signals of some sort that are hints the brain provides for a specific situation. The task is to recognize the signals and figuring out what they mean, but not let our feelings and emotions interfere with the decision-making process, in such an instance. They often cloud the decision-making process, which leads to making a wrong decision. This frequently happens in financial planning when individuals get caught up in the thought of getting rich. Their emotions misled them, and they lost massive amounts of money. Look at the many professional athletes who have made many millions and have gone broke.

Serendipitous

A serendipitous event is experiencing a favorable or beneficial outcome when it was never expected. We often try and plan everything and expect the outcomes to happen. Yet often an unplanned event happens, and completely redirects our living process. The reaction for most is to fight this change, which often leads to much frustration and anger. It is common for many people to say: why me? Yet, our frustration and unhappiness continue, until we accept the new reality. Often, when we get to acceptance, learn to manage our feelings, and move on with life, we will realize that the unplanned event has produced a positive outcome. Perhaps, the universe, a higher being, and or God, intervened, and redirected our plan, which puts us on the journey we were meant to be on. I do not have any other explanation, but it does happen.

Common Sense

A strong argument can be made that most people from 10 years old and up, lack common sense. Common sense is making a good judgement based on a simple perception of a situation.

I believe that common sense is a learned skill that is the result of problem-solving, which involves several steps of thinking: 1st) identifying simple options to a situation, 2nd) identifying potential outcomes to a situation based upon the options identified, and 3rd) identifying potential consequences of each option. People with common sense can mentally process a situation and produce an effective solution. It requires a sophisticated level of thinking that is learned early on from engaging in problem solving situations. Today, most people lack this skill because they have lacked situations to learn how to problem solve. Parents can help their children to learn skills for problem solving, which will help them in their adult life. However, many people are just too lazy to think a little harder and want others to problem solve for them. Developing common sense and learning to use it for problem solving, can really help our decision-making process. Specifically, this can help to prevent a lot of stress and frustration, which we can all do with less. Living becomes less complicated.

Presently, young adults and adults in general are very smart. That is, they may know a great deal about computers, math or other subject areas, but are lacking wisdom and common sense. Unfortunately, most people will never develop wisdom, or at least not much of it because they are becoming dependent upon artificial intelligence to do their thinking for them. Wisdom seems to be a combination of basic knowledge, our experiences, and incorporating our thoughts from our imagination. This combination expands one's consciousness, which creates a larger picture of the life we know and experience, and with what we don't know. Thus, the result is wisdom.

Such an individual who has these attributes seems to be well centered, at peace, comfortable with who they are, and seem to have things in order. In other words, their thinking process works very efficiently, as it connects all the knowledge available in the little rooms and pulling wisdom from the unconscious and the collective unconscious. Developing wisdom is also related to patience, thinking about events and experiences, in relation to what they feel, what they have learned, and how that leads to being a better person. There seems to be a connection/harmony between the inner sense of self, the consciousness, and the unconscious. A critical variable that incorporates these features is the imagination, which takes our thinking beyond the physical plain. Sometimes, many years will pass before wisdom is acquired from a past event, but only if one chooses to re-examine the experience, and seeks to learn a lesson that was not learned.

Perhaps, wisdom is a byproduct of common sense and could be developed from learning lessons from our experiences. However, most lessons learned come from our painful experiences, if we can manage the emotional pain. However, when an individual operates with a flawed emotional system, they are unable to effectively process powerful feelings and emotions that surface during painful experiences. Unfortunately, they will not learn the valuable lessons from the event, most likely, live in a constant state of anger, which hinders their thinking process and decision-making process. Another thought is maybe some people are born with a higher level of consciousness than most people, which seems to give them an edge in realizing a much larger picture of life. It seems when an individual has wisdom and common sense, they will be on a higher level of consciousness.

Consequently, they will experience less stress and emotional misery because they are better equipped to effectively manage difficult periods. However, for most people, the brain/thinking process does not work well when one will experience a significant loss/change event because their reality becomes a shattered reality. It is like a sudden storm that comes out of nowhere and catches us unprepared. Thinking with logic and reason is gone and taking its place is chaos, confusion, and anger.

Consequences of a malfunctioning thinking process controlled by anger include: domestic violence or any violence, going on a shopping spree, and spending vast amounts of money, taking drugs we would never have taken before, suddenly quitting our job, buying a new car, or something that the next day or week, you would say: why did I do this? Another crazy decision is to get married on the rebound. Have you ever been at a wedding ceremony, and when the couple are at the altar, you say to yourself: this marriage doesn't have a chance to make it. You know it, but the couple do not see it, or don't want to admit to this because they see what they want to see and not what is. Consequently, they are caught up in the moment. Have you ever done something out of the ordinary, and the next day you wake up and say: why did I do that? Clearly, your feelings and emotions at that moment caused your thinking process to malfunction. Slowing the mind down, either during the day, or at the end of the day, is a good thing to do. Create a silent sanctuary, maybe your bedroom, light a candle, lay down on the bed, and let your mind stop thinking. Let it take a break from processing and including some deep breathing exercises can be very beneficial. Plus, it is a great way to unwind, to lower your blood pressure, to escape the madness of the world and to bring your energy into harmony. One final thing to do, don't watch the news.

I don't what to call all these things, but what makes sense is that they are tools provided by our brain, or a higher power, which helps us to make good decisions. Decisions that help us to effectively manage the highs and lows of living, and to stay on the spiritual journey. I do not have a good explanation as why some people have these tools and others do not. My best guess is that people who do not have them are misguided by their feelings and emotions that override their ability to tap into their wisdom. Consequently, they grow little consciously, or not at all, and are denied the opportunity to connect to these tools, which can help make better decisions that can help keep the spiritual journey alive.

Chapter 3: An Ineffective Thinking Process

A lifelong task is to fine tune our thinking process, which will benefit our decision-making process, and lead to better outcomes. Failure to do so will lead to bad decision-making, which inhibits our ability to experience meaning, purpose, love, and hope. We do not live well without these attributes and are left with mood altering behaviors that lead to a troubled living process, which suffocates the human spirit. The process of fine tuning our thinking process, especially during a crisis, will expand our consciousness and reality. If expansion does not happen, one can become dominated by anger, which paralyzes our thinking process, which often leads to more anger and depression. Think of fine tuning your thinking process as being like taking your car in for a tune up because it is not running smoothly. The same principle applies to fine tuning our thinking process for creating an effective thinking process. Changing our thinking process and

belief system is no easy task because most people really want to hang on to their belief system because it creates a reality they know and feel comfortable with. However, our belief system is constantly being challenged by advances made in the scientific community, and by significant life changing events. For example, the science community created a vaccination that can immunized an individual from getting and dying from the virus, which can save your life. Yet, many Americans have not taken the vaccination because of a flawed thinking process that says no, and a lot of people have died that did not have to. This is the power of denial, a warped consciousness, and a flawed thinking process.

Currently, the country is being inundated with misinformation, which is confusing as to what is real and not real. This in turn challenges everyone's definition of meaning and purpose of their everyday experiences because this misinformation will threaten existing beliefs. For instance, Galileo told the world that the earth was not the center of the universe, and the pope ordered him to be put under house arrest for eight years, for making this statement. The church resisted this new concept because it threatened their ideology and limited reality because both provided power and control over people. Plus, it is easier to see what you want to see, especially when it serves your purpose. We often do the same thing. We resist what is true because it is easier to defend and protect our ineffective belief system, even if it causes suffering. This is what happens when the ego takes over the thinking process. This recently happened in Alabama. The supporters of Roy Moore voted for him because they saw what they wanted to see. However, they overlooked the fact that Moore has a history of not supporting and protecting the constitution, which is his primary responsibility, in addition to his other issues.

An especially important part of our thinking process is our mindset, which is comprised of a set of beliefs that lead to a personal philosophy. This, in turn, creates a specific reality. There are all kinds of individual realities, and we make decisions according to our reality. There are many realities, there is the republican and the democrat's view of the world. There is the Catholic view, the Muslim view, view of Buddhism, and the Mormon view, are a few additional views. Wealthy people have a vastly different view of the world, as compared to the view of poor people. People who have addictions see the world differently than people who do not have addictions. Furthermore, most people have difficulty to think well when experiencing a significant life changing event, which leads to reactive thinking.

The problem is that if one's reality is inaccurate/outdated, one becomes out of touch with what is really going on in their world and the larger world. This is a distorted reality, and often leads to discrimination, harassment, and behaviors related to ignorance. In essence, people see what they want to see, and this becomes a false reality because it does not match what is really going on in the bigger picture. Usually, this is not a good living process for the individual, and for others associated to this person because this determines their living process, which is dysfunctional. Sometimes people are so rigid in their thinking that they believe their beliefs guarantee specific outcomes. Outcomes as: life is fair, our children will turn out, and love and happiness happen, once we make money, get married, and become successful. Many people live believing these experiences are guaranteed when in fact nothing is guaranteed. It is a huge mistake to believe otherwise because frustration and anger will be the outcome. An example has been the people who did not believe in the covet vaccination, which could have protected them. Many such individuals got the virus, and many died, when death could have been prevented.

Our thinking process is also influenced by various filters that create our reality, which include money, physical beauty, politics, religion, type of car one drives, ethnicity, and color are a few. These factors influence our thinking process, and our decision-making process, often in a negative way. This is like looking at a beautiful looking cake, tasting the frosting and loving it, but then you take a bite of the cake and hate it. Another example is judging a book by its cover. Our filters do the same thing because we do not see the entire picture, but often see what we want to see. Furthermore, a flawed self-definition will automatically create a flawed thinking process because we see the world in relation to how we see our self. An individual with a severe flawed sense of self will often see the world as a scary place, and approach living with fear, and a lack of confidence. However, others may have an inflated ego, and try to overrun everyone in their path, which never produces anything good. An ineffective thinking process will create a distorted reality that leads to bad decision-making, bad outcomes, and a troubled living process.

Eventually, bad decision-making leads to a dead end because the misery and suffering becomes a 24/7 experience, and the misery becomes overwhelming because people lose hope. Some individuals who want to create a healthy lifestyle often seek therapy because they do not know the cause of their dysfunctional behavior, nor know how, or what to change, but they know they are experiencing a troubled living process. A positive change occurs when a therapist helps the patient address their unresolved emotional core issues, which frees them from their emotional prison because the healing process brings the repressed feeling from the unconscious to the conscious. From here, the patient can process these powerful feelings and not let them influence our thinking process. Consequently, one will begin to experience wholeness and harmony, and begin to create a healthy self-definition. In addition, they will also begin to examine their belief system. The result is an improved thinking process that creates a renewed sense of purpose, meaning and hope that life can and will get better because they have a more accurate picture of reality.

Presently, many people have a thinking process that reflects the cultural norms of society that feeling good for the moment, or just do it, is what is important. Little thinking is required. Sadly, this is their reality and their reference point for decision-making, which is guided by raw feelings and emotions instead of logic and reason. Thus, a messy troubled living process. Furthermore, today there is very little structure that guides us through our decision-making, which gives way to people living with a moment to moment mentally. This type of mentality originates from a flawed thinking process that has little restraint and reacts to emotional impulses. Sadly, such an individual will often sacrifice a bright future because over time, our bad decision making will catch up to us. Just ask Matt Lauer, Harvey Weinstein, Tiger Woods, Charlie Rose, and Bill Gates. In the end, their troubled living process got out of control, which led to a variety of problems and life changing events.

Flawed Reality: A Flawed Thinking Process
An ineffective reality begins to formulate when there is a disordered relationship between the conscious and the unconscious, which gives birth to a flawed self–definition, flawed emotional system and flawed mindset. The accumulative interaction creates a flawed thinking process that leads to a distorted reality and bad decision-making that creates a troubled living process.

Flawed Thinking Process

| Flawed Self Definition | + | Flawed Emotional System | + | Flawed Mindset | = | Flawed Decision Making |

The cornerstone of our flawed thinking process is a flawed self-definition, which is caused from growing up in a toxic family environment. The result is the formation of a shame-based self-definition. Specifically, feelings of being inadequate will dominate such an individual, which leads to a disordered relationship between the conscious and the unconscious. This gives way to an automatic creation of a flawed emotional system and a flawed mindset. A flawed thinking process is now in place, which leads to bad decision-making with bad outcomes.

Flawed Self-Definition (FSD)
The concept of dysfunction (Friel & Friel, 1988) is well documented. This begins with a flawed self-definition that resonates from growing up in a toxic environment that leads to a shame-

based self-definition. This becomes the cornerstone for a flawed thinking process. Think of a cake recipe. You make the cake, but forgot to include an important ingredient, and the cake does not turn out the way it is supposed to. Love, a sense of security, and a sense of predictability are essential ingredients for a healthy development of self. When these ingredients are insufficient or totally missing, especially during the first year of life, the result is a flawed self-definition. A child will always know when they are not loved, or when mom or dad have their issues that become more important than the child. The world of a child is exceedingly small, and mainly consist of their interaction with their parents and the environment created by their parents. Children crave their parent's love, which is measured by the commitment of time and energy the parents give to the child. The child will know when they do not receive enough love, it is an unconscious reaction that happens automatically. In addition, the child automatically represses the painful feelings into the unconscious, which begins the disordered relationship between the conscious and the unconscious. Sadly, this gives birth to the child's flawed self-definition and the development of a flawed thinking process.

Without sufficient love, the experience of shame begins in infancy. An infant/child will lack cognitive skills to process any experience but is able to detect painful anti-love messages. Think of a time you were in a meeting, on a date, or at some interaction with others, and just felt uncomfortable. You were picking up some sort of signal/vibes about how you did not fit in this situation. Infants can also detect these messages, which come in various forms. Verbal abuse is the most common form of anti-love and is often experienced when caring adults make statements as: you're stupid, dumb, or screaming, and/or scolding a child. Criticizing is a very damaging practice because it creates a sense of shame. It sends the message to the child that they are flawed and defective because they are unable to live up to the expectations of the parents. Another destructive verbal practice is when a child is constantly being put down. Call your child dumb or stupid enough times, and they will believe what you tell them. Then there is physical abuse as slapping and striking the child. Not only does this cause physical pain, but also give the message that the child is not a valued human being, nor worthy of good things. Consequently, they will internalize these messages in a negative way, which leads to the formation of a flawed self-definition.

In addition, are parents who frequently argue, or verbally fight, create a toxic environment of fear, anxiety, and distrust, and the child will have issues of trusting anyone, nor feel worthy or valued. At some time, the child may even feel responsible for the parental conflict, which reinforces their belief that they are flawed and defective and not worthy of love. Parents who create extremely strict boundaries or totally lack boundaries are also guilty of not providing adequate love because parents confuse having control or not having any control, is a form of allowing total freedom or having no freedom, as love, when it is not. Providing rules and some discipline for children shows you care and love them, which is an especially important message. Furthermore, a child will always know when parents do not love them because they can sense the sincerity of the message.

There are also non-behavioral forms of abuse such as when parents ignore their infant for extended periods of time or ignore the baby even when the child is in distress. These are perceived as anti-love messages. In large families, the youngest child may suffer from anti-love messages because parents are often tired of raising kids, and they just do not provide enough quality loving time. Other powerful events include divorce when children are in their formative years, or when dad or mom is absent, like serving in the military for an extended period of time, or if a parent dies. The child may feel responsible for these events and conclude they are unlovable.

Another behavior that has a negative impact on a child's development, is if either mom or dad suffers from addictions, or have serious mental health issues such as chronic depression. In both situations the parent(s) is not emotionally available for the child. Then there are parents who use the child to fulfill their own emotional needs, which is very damaging because the child does not have anything to give because they do not have much of a sense of self. The result is that the child's sense of self becomes underdeveloped, which is a set up for a flawed self-definition. The most damaging anti-love message is sexual abuse, which is a profoundly serious societal problem that usually goes undetected because the victim does not want to talk about it. In this form of abuse, the person the child trusted and assumed would protect them from harm, created the harm. This has a devastating impact on the child's sense of self, their ability to trust, and their ability to develop and maintain healthy loving relationships. Furthermore, this child will seek dysfunctional relationships that are always a painful experience, which never end well. In addition, if family turmoil is severe, and other experiences as rape, incest, and other traumatic events are experienced, the individual will experience core trauma, which results in extreme damage to our psychological inner sense of self that are often repressed deep within our unconscious and will severely alter one's self-definition and thinking process.

Consequently, the child will not see themselves as being worthy of love, have great difficulty in loving themselves, and anyone else. The result of the parent's neglect is the perception of shame, guilt, and a deep feeling of insecurity because these become the dominating factors that influence and form one's flawed self-definition. Shame is experienced as a deep feeling of being flawed and defective, is toxic to the development of self, and to the human spirit because it prevents a child from becoming whole and healthy. A child or infant is unable to manage these painful feelings but know when they are not loved. Overtime, they develop the belief they are not loveable, or not worthy of love, which gives birth to a flawed self-definition. This becomes an exceptionally large handicap that creates a messy troubled living process because we try and do things to make up for this lack of love, but this approach only creates additional emotional problems because there is no substitute for love.

The child with a flawed self-definition will then develop a fractured ego that will direct their thinking process, which never goes well. Most decisions are an attempt to satisfy their insecurities and inner sense of emptiness. Decision-making is guided by the need to be validated by others, the need for power, and or control, to be accepted, to use others for their own gain, and rescuing others. As a result, many individuals create an identity as a by-product of their fractured ego and identify themselves with their ego. For instance, whatever your job title is, you perform according to the rules of behavior defined by that title, but this creates a problem, if you perform and act the same way when you are home with your family and loved ones. Most people have many identities and being healthy implies that we learn to live effectively with all our identities. This can help to simplify living process and enjoyable because we experience fewer problems and the stress that accompanies them.

Think for a second and recall an event when you did something you wish you had not. How did you feel the next day? Did you look in the mirror and not like what you saw? This is shame and when we have a flawed self-definition, we experience continuous shame because we have a flawed or scarred inner core, and believe we are never good enough. In addition, we pile on more shame when we make bad decisions that only creates the wrong experience. In addition, we often ignore and repress our painful feelings deep within the unconscious. Consequently, these painful feelings never really disappear, but continue to fester and silently influence our thinking process, which leads to bad decision-making and bad outcomes. Thus, a troubled living experience. If our childhood was extremely painful, one can bury/repress their painful feelings so deep that one cannot recall or remember the event that caused them. This is a profoundly serious issue that needs to be addressed by a professional therapist.

Left to fester within, shame will accumulate and often manifest as a gnawing feeling, which we often believe is caused by being over stressed, or maybe we ate something that upset our stomach. This gnawing feeling goes away but is still active and reappears every now and then. Eventually, this inner churning pain creates an imbalance within the depths of our psychological inner core, and disrupts our thinking process, which begins to become controlled by addictive thinking. Sexually abused individuals will have an imbalance within their psychological inner core, often eat their way through this pain, and the result is significant weight gain. This is often a defense mechanism, that is, no one will find them to be sexually attractive. The accumulative affect is the creation of a flawed sense of self that leads to a flawed thinking process that results in bad decision-making that is about coping. The result is a destructive troubled living process that is known as co-dependency.

Co-dependency is a common disorder. In its broadest sense, co-dependency is an addiction to people, behaviors, or things. In short, it is the need to be needed, which is an addiction. Co-dependency is about the fallacy of trying to control interior feelings by controlling people, things, and events. To the co-dependent, control, or the lack of it, is central to every aspect of life (Hemfelt, Minirth, & Meier, 1989). Co-dependents become like vacuum cleaners gone wild drawing to themselves not just to another person, but also chemicals, usually alcohol, and other drugs, or things such as money, food sports, sex, and gambling or even work. They struggle relentlessly to fill the intense sense of emptiness within themselves, but never do (Hemfelt, Minirth, & Meier, 1989).

The efforts of the co-dependent are about trying to fill a deep inner void, which manifest as a flawed self-definition. This was created from growing up in a dysfunctional toxic family. The constant helping others provides some self-validation, a sense of power, and control, and instant positive feedback from others, which often becomes their drug. Please understand that not everyone who is helping others is suffering from co-dependency. We need to live with compassion, and always help others in need, but not to the point that we lose our sense of self, and or our loved ones. Realize that the rescuer always becomes the victim, and this can lead to serious health problems. Our dysfunction may also manifest as the over achiever, the family hero, the family clown, and the people pleaser (Hemfelt, Minirth, & Meier, 1989). All of these reflects a deep inner core problem that becomes a flawed self-definition, and a flawed thinking process.

Furthermore, many of a co-dependent's compulsions and addictions, such as alcoholism, drug abuse, and eating disorders are also life threatening. Rage and physical abuse are also traits of co-dependents and can endanger the lives of innocents (Hemfelt, Minirth, & Meier, 1989). The emotional impact touches all their loved ones. Without healthy coping strategies, they also become emotionally overwhelmed, and get pushed to rely on destructive mood-altering behaviors. The cause is a flawed thinking process that was the result of unresolved core feelings that created the flawed self-definition.

The Ten Traits of a Co-dependent (Hemfelt, Minirth & Meier, 1989)
1. The co-dependent is driven by one or more compulsions.
2. The co-dependent is bound and often tormented by the way things were in family of origin.
3. The co-dependent's self-esteem (and frequently maturity) is exceptionally low.
4. A co-dependent is certain his or her happiness hinges on others.
5. Conversely, a co-dependent feels inordinately responsible for others.
6. The co-dependent's relationship with a spouse, or significant other, is marred by a damaging unstable lack of balance between dependence and independence.
7. The co-dependent is a master of denial and repression.
8. The co-dependent worries about things he or she can't change and may well try and change them.
9. A co-dependent's life is punctuated by extremes.
10. A co-dependent is constantly looking for the something that is missing or lacking in life.

Other Characteristics of Co-dependency (Hemfelt, Minirth & Meier, 1989)
1. Live by denial.
2. Full of anger, most of it is hidden and unsuspected.
3. Get love confused with intensity and romantic feelings.

4. Must manipulate or control others.
5. They have few or no boundaries.
6. Full of self-hate.
7. Always have a feeling of chronic emptiness.
8. They repress their feelings and become numb.
9. The emotional pain within continues to fester and grow.
10. They look for a fix to alleviate the emotional pressure.
11. Tremendous emotional pressure builds that eventually explodes.
12. Greatest fear is abandonment and rejection.
13. In the advanced stages, a common symptom is relationship addiction. They must have a relationship, which is like a drink is to an alcoholic.
14. In the advanced stages, addictions develop along with compulsive behaviors.

Life and Co-dependency
Co-dependency is an unhealthy troubled living process that causes erosion of our sense of self because our existence is dependent upon pleasing others and taking care of others. Consequently, we fail to nurture ourselves because we often get used and manipulated. In time, we become dependent upon others to validate our sense of self, which becomes a set up for a troubled living process. Furthermore, losing control of one's thinking process is a major characteristic of co-dependency. The healthy life becomes a fading dream regardless of how the individual attempts to manipulate people and objects. It can even result in death because physical health will often deteriorate and gives way to serious health problems. It can also result in suicide because life may totally spin out of control because purpose, meaning, love, and hope are severely diminished.

Interpretation of Events
Misinterpretation of events is common among co-dependents because of their inaccurate reality and flawed thinking process. Failed experiences are often magnified, often perceived as rejection, and feeling inadequate, which reinforces our flawed self-definition. Consider the following experiences.

* You are trying out for the soccer team. However, you are not very good, you get cut from the team, or you remain on the team, but never play.
* You're planning to ask someone out for a date, and you get the courage to ask, but he/she says no.
* You have experienced one bad relationship after another.
* You don't get that promotion and wonder why?
* You have a job interview, but don't get the job.
* You take a test and get a bad grade.

Experiences of failure and rejection are common in our living process and they hurt. However, they should not reflect, nor reinforce the perception that one is flawed and defective. However, because we are living with a flawed thinking process, our misinterpretation highlights our **perceived inadequacies** that include the following.

* I am not smart enough.
* I am not tall enough.
* There must be something wrong with me.
* I am not good looking.
* I am not the right color.
* No one loves me.
* No one thinks I am important.
* No one cares about me.
* No one likes me.
* I always fail at what I do.
* I can't do anything right.

If we constantly have these thoughts, we will become what we think! We must stop thinking these bad thoughts! This only reinforces our already existing flawed self-definition. In fact, it will make it worse. The reaction to failure and rejection often becomes a learned response that may stay with us throughout our life. **Not a good thing!** When we have a flawed thinking process and experience failure we often create the following **negative feelings**.

* Fear and shame.
* Rage and being afraid.
* Jealousy and loneliness.
* Self-pity and being sad.
* Being inferior and feeling hurt.
* Feeling insecure.
* Feel like we are not good enough.

These negative feelings are very powerful, often stay with us, and produce the following **conclusions**.

Conclusions
* A feeling of hopelessness.
* A feeling of self-condemnation.
* A feeling of powerlessness.
* Believing we are a victim.
* Believing that everyone is against me.
* Want others to make me happy.

This flawed thinking process only reinforces our existing flawed self-definition. Instead of living with self-confidence and pursuing dreams, we become consumed with low expectations and live with a lack of self–confidence. However, others become the over achievers, or the family hero, or a people pleaser, or the family clown (Hemfelt, Minirth, & Meier, 1989). Their attempts or accomplishments are efforts to get them noticed, accepted, and provides some degree of validation. However, the inner pain is not healed, and will still haunt their decision-making. Furthermore, we all have defenses to protect our deep insecurities, which is fuel for sustaining our troubled living process. Unknowingly, our accomplishments are often attempts to fill our inner emptiness caused by the lack of love from growing up in a toxic family.

A Flawed self-definition will also manifest as having ineffective boundaries. Some will live with fragile boundaries and have difficulty in saying no because they have an inner need to be validated and accepted by others because they are unable to love themselves. This often results in being used and manipulated, and anger will eventually be the result. Others will have rigid boundaries and believe they have everything figured out because they have all the answers. They become the self-righteous, opinionated, and function as judge and executioner. They see what they want to see and not what is because control is their main goal. Sadly, this has become the extreme right wing, and their only goal is obtaining power. Anyone who enters this environment will have to give up their control and accept the reality that is provided.

A flawed self-definition will also be the cause of our character flaws that interfere with our decision-making process. For instance, often our weaknesses are strengths overdone. It is wonderful to be trusting, but this becomes a problem when we trust too much. It is wonderful to love, but this becomes a problem when one loves too much. These are character flaws that influence our decision-making process that often result in bad outcomes that cause a lot of emotional suffering.

The following is a list of behaviors that often-become character flaws that contribute to making bad decisions that lead to emotional suffering. Using the 1 to 5 scale, provide a score for each. This will provide a degree of how your character flaws are controlling your life.

Don't like
Like too much _____

Don't work
Work too much _____

Don't spend
Spend too much _____

Don't watch TV
Watch too much TV _____

Don't drink
Drink too much _____

Don't exercise
Exercise too much _____

Don't feel
Feel too much _____

Don't talk
Talk too much _____

Don't please
Please too much _____

Eat a little
Eat too much _____

Don't worry
Worry too much _____

Don't play
Play too much _____

Don't trust
Trust too much _____

No dependency
Too much dependency _____

No control
Too much control _____

No thinking
Thinking too much _____

Not enough money
Too much money _____

No emotional pain
Too much emotional pain _____

Very little sensitivity
Too much sensitivity _____

No self-love
Too much self-love _____

No arguing
Too much arguing _____

Total = _____

Divide the total by 21. If your overall score is near 5 or 1, your decision-making is controlled by character flaws that reflect a flawed self-definition. This is a flawed thinking process that diminishes one's self-definition because such a person is making bad decisions that often erode their sense of self. Stop and think for a second of what kind of life you want to live? Do you want to live with a flawed thinking process that erodes your sense of self that leads to bad decision-making and emotional misery?

Some of us grew up in a healthy family environment and have few unresolved emotional core issues, or at least not serious enough to address. However, we have survived childhood, but not without some psychological scars caused from anti-love messages from our toxic family. The result is a flawed self-definition that becomes the cornerstone of our flawed thinking process. Sadly, the real self is in hiding, waiting to rise to the surface, and then we can become who we were meant to be. Until we discover our real self, we do not even know who we are, let others define us, and we often act, and live according to a role defined by someone else, or institutional rules, or religious rules. In addition, a common outcome is to get into relationships that are very dysfunctional, which always lead to a bad experience. This flawed thinking process creates a false reality, which leads to bad decision-making. The development of a flawed self-definition gives birth to a flawed emotional system.

Flawed Emotional System
Feelings are real, and they matter. Stop for a moment, and go back in your history, and do the following: How far back in your life can you go, and remember when someone hurt your feelings? I bet it was quite early in your life. The point is that painful feelings stay with us, and when we stop and think about the event that caused the painful feelings, we can even get choked up about it. What movie made you cry? Why? Feelings are what makes us feel alive, and we love it when we have positive feelings. However, painful feelings are also powerful, and we don't like to feel miserable, at least not for very long. A flawed emotional system will enhance our pain, and then we look for a quick fix of some sort.
Furthermore, long term repressed feelings can have harmful effects on the body, and influence

how one lives their life. It acts as a powerful silent rip tide that quietly messes with the flow of life. During times of experiencing intense short-term feelings, some people may not sleep much, or use eating as a coping strategy, or do not eat much at all, or engage in some other destructive behavior. We have all experienced bad painful feelings caused, usually by a loved one. For instance, most people believe that verbal abuse and physical abuse do not cause any lasting harm. These are very destructive behaviors that create painful feelings and emotions that can lead to despair, anger, and sometimes hopelessness. Physical abuse can also lead to living with extreme fear, and have a harmful effect on our self-definition, which is always a dreadful experience.

Unexpressed feelings and emotions will become a major problem because they can dominate the living landscape by influencing our thinking process. Furthermore, we lack skills to effectively manage our painful feelings and emotions, and the result is making decisions without logic, or reason. The result is an impulsive decision-making process that cause unnecessary emotional suffering. The un-intendent consequence is to rely on bad decision-making to engage in some form of mood-altering behavior. Instead of life getting better, life gets worse, but our mood altering does provides some short-term relief. This becomes a vicious cycle, which often defines a troubled life, however, most people put on a happy face to hide their misery, while they quietly engage in some mood-altering behavior.

Then there are life changing events, which most people will experience and are a significant loss/change experience. The emotional fallout can be so painful that they really do re-arrange our thinking process and living experiences. That is, extreme stress overwhelms the individual's belief system and their emotional system, which is unable to effectively process the powerful feelings and emotions. The result is a distorted reality, which creates total confusion. The individual does not know what is up or down because their raw feelings and emotions change their reality by the moment. Consequently, many people get lost in their thinking process and are vulnerable to making many bad decisions. Unfortunately, their living process breaks down and purpose, meaning, and hope are diminished. Instead of being creative and find ways to cope, and to make sense out of the life changing event, the individual's flawed thinking process automatically goes to self-pity.

Self-pity is a state of mind, in which the individual's thinking process becomes incapacitated because they feel sorry for themselves. Thoughts as: I did not deserve this, life isn't fair, and there must be something wrong with me, I can't do anything right, and then sometimes they have the thought as how to seek revenge. These thoughts erode our sense of hope, and many people give up. That is, depression and anger have won because they have paralyzed the thinking process. These thoughts of self-pity occur because the individual becomes overcome with extreme grief, depression, and anger, which their flawed emotional system and flawed thinking process are unable to effectively manage. These are thoughts that paralyze the thinking process, and sometimes, for a lifetime, which means the outcome is a life of misery.

Yes, some grief and depression are normal with the occurrence of life changing events, but it is not normal when they immobilize one's thinking process for a lifetime.

A friend committed suicide because of not being able to manage a stressful life event. Consequently, self-pity thinking overwhelmed his thinking process, and instantly took him to a deep state of depression and anger, and to a reactionary decision to commit suicide. How sad! His children needed him! His thinking process failed him because he could not see that his children were more important than him committing suicide. He did not have to commit suicide. All he had to do was to change his thinking, but self-pity prevented this from happening. His emotional system and flawed thinking process failed him. Do not get me wrong, one gets to be angry when a bad thing happens, but only for a short time because anything beyond is a waste of energy and time. Furthermore, decisions made by anger never lead to a good solution, in fact most anger related decisions will only increase our misery and make things worse for our loved ones.

A flawed emotional system is created when we grow up in a family that is rich in emotional turmoil that becomes the source of anti-love messages. Painful messages include the same behaviors discussed in the previous chapter. However, another important source comes from needy parents, and when parents have addictions. Their own needs become more important than the needs of the child and they are unable to create a loving environment. The child can sense when they are not loved and believe something is wrong with them because if they were perfect, mom and dad would spend more time with them. This rejection is very painful, and this will also create and reinforce a flawed self-definition. Furthermore, the child lacks the ability to manage these painful feelings. The only thing they can do is to repress them into their unconscious, which only comes back to haunt them by messing with the thinking process.

As we get a little older and begin to participate in sports, we will experience an injury and are often told to block out the pain and play through it. Think of how many times we have witnessed athletes, at all levels, play through their injuries and admire them for doing so. Then there are times during childhood when boys will cry and are told by an adult that big boys do not cry. The message is given that crying is a sign of weakness, and boys do not want others to see them as a weakling. Being unemotional is seen as being tough, which is valued by society. People entering the military are also programmed not to feel, and the intention is to keep on mission, and not to become incapacitated by painful feelings and emotions.

Furthermore, a soldiers' survival may be determined by not feeling. Soldiers often experience traumatic adrenalin filled experiences that are never to be experienced by the average citizen. Even thou a soldier participates in extensive training; they are not prepared emotionally for the reality of death and destruction that occurs in war. This leaves one course of action, which is to repress intense feelings and emotions that destroys the integrity of the emotional system, and often, their belief system. They then return home, and their repressed feelings and ineffective emotional system malfunctions, as does their thinking process, which leads to post-traumatic stress. This interferes with their ability to create meaning, purpose, love, and hope. Consequently, they become very confused. To cope with this failure, they usually engage in destructive behaviors that only cause more confusion and misery that can lead to suicide. Presently, approximately 22 veterans commit suicide every day.

Furthermore, males in general are not emotionally available. Ask a guy what he is feelings, and he will usually respond by saying, "I don't know", or just not say anything because he isn't feeling anything and doesn't know how to feel. Women tend to be more emotional than men, however, women are also learning to repress feeling and emotions because more are moving up in the work force and increasing their involvement in sports. A perceived emotional requirement in the work force and in sports is to have everything under control, including one's feelings. Like men, women are learning to repress feelings, and this often becomes the standard for the rest of their life, which also has a negative effect on other areas of their life. Growing up in a toxic environment children become emotionally unavailable. Furthermore, we learn by our experiences, and we don't often have many role models that provide healthy ways for effectively managing feelings and emotions. Overtime, our repressed feelings create an emotional volcano that is lacking an effective release valve. This is evident when the reaction to an event is way out of proportion to the act that caused the reaction. For example, a friend accidently spills your coffee, and you react by punching him, or screaming at him. To say the least, your friend probably won't want to be your friend anymore, and he/she will have difficulty trusting you again.

The minor event of spilling the coffee unleashed built up feelings that have been festering for a very long time from the constant practice of repressing them. The person overreacted because it is a normal response when one is emotionally overloaded. Furthermore, an individual has unresolved emotional issues, whenever a reaction is out of proportion to an event, such as the above example. Many violent acts occur because of an automatic over reaction to some minor infraction caused by a flawed emotional system. Tuck the following thought in your conscious mind: the hardest thing to do in a crisis is "nothing."

Repressed feelings will also create an overloaded emotional system that will disrupt energy flow, which also stresses the physiological systems. This in turn can compromise the immune system, and over time, one can become vulnerable to disease and illness. I believe a friend died of cancer because he had a flawed emotional system. That is, his physiological systems were overloaded because of a lifetime of built-up unexpressed emotions and feelings. He was unable to express his feelings and emotions, they piled up within the unconscious. Eventually, this caused his physiological systems to break down because of the stress caused by his negative energy stored within his unconscious, which led to cancer. Another product of a flawed emotional system are anxiety attacks. Repressed emotions and feelings build up and without notice, erupt, and cognitively, for a period, one is unable to process information, and function appropriately.

It is not an accident we become emotionally flawed and defective. Its creation is automatic when one grows up in a family rich in emotional turmoil. A child will grow up with fear and anxiety because they fear expressing their feelings and emotions. Consequently, they develop a flawed self-definition and a flawed emotional system because of anti-love messages. The best a child can do is to repress these painful feelings, unfortunately, they learn this method of emotional management and perfect it. This flawed emotional system fails to efficiently identify, express, and process painful feelings and emotions. Furthermore, we will also lack the ability to experience closure with painful life changing events, which prevents one from moving on in a positive way. In essence, our flawed emotional system fuels the flawed thinking process, and the result is bad decision making.

Flawed Mindset (FMS)
A FMS is the final variable that shapes our thinking process. A FMS is comprised of individual faulty beliefs that are assumptions that often become expectations that forms our consciousness/reality. We always make decisions according to our reality, which is a problem when we have a distorted reality. For example, my father died in his early sixties, and for many years, out of anger, my mother would often say: it was not fair that he died so young. Her mindset was comprised of the following beliefs: she believed that going to church every Sunday, turning the other cheek, being overly humble, work hard, always helping others, believing God would take care of everything, all things would work out, and they would live to be old. In her thinking, life should be fair, and living to be old was guaranteed. However, my dad died before he got old, and therefore, she believed life was unfair, and the only emotional outcome from this is anger. Please understand that anger is a normal experience when something does not work out the way we expect it to, or if a life changing event happens unexpectedly. However, anger is not normal nor healthy when it consumes us and controls our thinking because it will sabotage all aspects of our life. Anger will resonate throughout every aspect of our living process and have a negative impact on how we live. Anger is always the enemy to healthy change because it paralyzes the thinking process.

Our painful, and happy feelings influence the decisions we make, and how we interpret experiences in relation to our reality. The mindset is like a computer that processes information. The problem occurs when we have a mindset that creates a distorted reality because we process experiences according to our reality. It is like having the wrong computer software. A FMS will lead to the misinterpretation of life, in general, and life experiences, which will produce more frustration, fear, anxiety, and anger, that sometimes will last a lifetime. Furthermore, these can become extremely intense and lead to drastic mood-altering behaviors, or some people just give up and live within their depression. The individual with a FMS will have poor coping methods, which will lead to poor decision-making and a troubled living process. Collectively, the following beliefs create a FMS that will create an inaccurate reality that will misinterpret life events.

Modern Flawed Mindset
* Feeling good is happiness.
* Social status is most important.
* He/she will make me happy.
* Bad things won't happen to me.
* I am indestructible.
* I will live forever.
* Money will buy happiness.
* Children will provide my happiness.
* We will live happily ever after.
* Happiness is having sex appeal, money, and power.
* Happiness is a new house.
* Happiness is a sporty car.
* My career will provide my happiness.
* Pain and suffering is an unnecessary element of life.
* I can control the uncontrollable.
* Others will make me happy.
* Life is fair.
* Love is an easy thing to do.
* I don't need an education.
* Relationships are not that difficult.
* I can change him or her.
* We will always look good.
* Nothing will get between us.
* Life is not difficult.
* I don't have to work hard to be successful.
* If I am loyal, loyalty will be return.
* What goes around never comes around.
* Things look better on the other side of the fence.
* We can never have enough things.
* All my problems would be gone, if I went someplace else.
* I am not responsible for my problems.
* I can do whatever I want.

A flawed mindset will create a distorted reality, which leads to bad decision making. Consequently, our flawed emotional system will be unable to effectively process painful feelings, which will then accumulate and create an over loaded emotional system. The next thing is to mood alter, which becomes an automatic response, and only makes living a more difficult experience. Elton John created a CD called The Big Picture that describes the pain of a

dysfunctional life in music. The dynamics of the dysfunctional life can also be seen in the following films.
* **Good Will Hunting**
* **Prince of Tides**
* **Bliss**

In essence, a troubled living process, but has become the norm in society. It's caused by unresolved emotional core issues lead to a disordered relationship between the conscious and the unconscious. This gives birth to a flawed thinking process, which is characterized by impulsive decision making guided by poorly managed feelings and emotions that lead to bad outcomes. The accumulative effect of bad decision-making caused by a flawed thinking process is toxic to the human spirit and gives way to the addictive personality. Mood altering is how most people numb their emotional misery from their troubled living process, and often they become addictions, and their misery escalates to a whole new level.

A troubled living process robs us from becoming who we were meant to become. It robs us from living the life we want. It robs us from creating healthy loving relationships. It robs us from having freedom of choice. It robs us from effectively living in society and from creating meaning, purpose, love, and hope.

Conflicted Thoughts
Conflicted thoughts are a product of a flawed thinking process, and they cause a lot of confusion and stress. Everyone has conflicted thoughts, for example, there are things that you like about your congressional representative, and things you do not like, there are things you like about your kids, and things you don't like, and there are things you like about your spouse, and things you don't like, and these are all normal. However, conflicting thoughts can cause serious stress and confusion when they dominate your thinking process. Like when you are thinking about a highly valued people in your life, and or things that are dear to you. Think of a loving relationship, in which you love your partner because he/she is caring, loving, and hardworking. Yet, their mismanagement of money makes you hate them or strongly dislike them. Another example is that your partner had an affair, and you love them and forgive them, but a part of you hates them for what they did. Maybe hate is too strong of a word, but strongly dislike is another word that can be used to describe the situation created by conflicted thoughts.

Conflicting thoughts create disharmony because the dominate feelings often are anger, dislike, and even hate, and these are very powerful and can destroy relationships. If not destroying them, then they will often create a less than loving situation and make the relationship exceedingly difficult. Both partners can feel these ill feelings because they become evident in our mannerisms, speech patterns, and other behaviors. They create a lot of uncertainty, which will lead to unhappiness, and if both partners are unable to resolve this distress, they will drift

54

apart. Conflicted thoughts, also cause disharmony within an individual because energy goes to each thought, which can lead to an energy drain, difficulty in sleeping, and difficulty in staying focused. We always function better when our mind, body, and sense of self have clarity and harmony.

Chapter 4: Creating an Effective Thinking Process

Creating an effective thinking process will help address the disordered relationship between the conscious and the unconscious, which will lead to wholeness. Healing old emotional wounds will help to create harmony and wholeness, which will allow one to create a healthy living process. More specifically, the beginning of creating a healthy self-definition, which becomes the cornerstone for a healthy thinking process. The following formula is comprised of the components that create an effective thinking process.

An Effective Thinking Process

Hlthy Self	+	Effective	+	Effective Mindset	+	Everyday Living	=	Life Outcome
Definition		Emotional		(Options, Tech Skills)		(Psych Needs)		Good Decisions
(integrity)		System		(Rules & Guidelines)		(Goals, Vision)		
(dignity)				(Essential EI, Beliefs)				

Happiness

The first task is to examine the concept of happiness and success, which are defined in many different ways. Most people never have given much thought about these two concepts. How we define them determines the direction of our living process. For instance, if an individual's focus is on making money, and buying the good life, but ignoring their sense of self, and failing to nurture significant loving relationships, then they may have the good life, but and empty life.

Happiness must include a love of self and having significant loving relationships, which requires having a healthy self-definition will lead to love and acts of love, which lead to purpose, meaning, and love. A flawed self-definition is a problem because I cannot love another because I am not able to give what I don't have, which is not being able to love oneself. Many people experience moments of feeling good, which often becomes a substitute for happiness. Most people have been programmed to believe that happiness are moments that produce feel good feelings and emotions, experienced when specific experiences happen. This has led us to become a feel-good society, and most people have little restraint in making decisions to feel good for the moment, but this is not happiness.

Furthermore, many people believe that the greater the discrepancy between what we have and what we want, the more unhappy we are. Many people have set a high bar for what they think will make them happy, which helps explain why people always want more because they are never satisfied with what they have. For instance, many people believe they must have that nice new expensive car, or truck, or a new modern house, the current trend for clothes and jewelry, the new expensive phones, and must take that expensive vacation every year, to be happy. The couple in Colorado had all these things, which created a great image, but beneath the surface was an entangled living mess with a huge financial problem, and the dad was having an affair. Despite this image of happiness and all is well image, dad murdered his wife and children. At some point in their living process, dad got misdirected by a flawed thinking process that failed to define and understand love, which led to this tragedy.

Furthermore, one can determine their happiness by identifying what they complain about. Generally, if you complain about little things, you don't have big problems. If you have big problems little problems do not matter. However, if you do not find the right solution for little problems, they might evolve into big problems. When our dysfunction is extreme, people will have a lot of big problems because they are always consumed by their crisis mode of thinking and are never satisfied, or happy. Furthermore, many individuals often get caught up in comparing their lives to others, and this is usually not a good thing to do because you are allowing others to define your image of the good life. Adolescents, frequently, compare themselves to their peers, which is a means to set the bar as to what is acceptable behavior. This comparison thinking often becomes a means for how they define themselves, which is not a good thing because they never measure up.

Realizing that your life could be a lot worse, and that many people have a life much worse than yours, is very important to realize. This helps one to create an accurate larger picture, which is important for the thinking that follows. In most instances, an unhappy person has not realized that happiness is much more than the acquisition of material things, but rather is about how one feels within, about how one feels about self, and how one defines themselves. Having order in one's life is also important for happiness because lacking order is about a life unraveling. Happiness is about looking in the mirror and liking who you are. Happiness and success are directly related to finding your passion, doing positive things for yourself, and for others, all of which helps make the world a better place. Also included is living with compassion and creating and maintaining loving relationships. Life is, also much easier when we make life simple. The accumulation of these experiences creates meaning, purpose, love and hope, which creates a healthier happy spiritual journey.

Happiness includes the following features
* Happiness is not walking around with a smile, but rather a sense of being at peace with who you are.
* Having a sense of inner peace and a feeling of wholeness and harmony.
* A sense of inner confidence.
* A sense of having order in life.
* Minimizing and preventing stressors and unnecessary stressful life events.
* Having healthy loving relationships.
* Having a healthy sense of purpose and meaning.
* The capability to nurture your sense of self by creating healthy boundaries.
* To function at a high level of consciousness.
* To grow spiritually.
* To live with kindness and compassion.

Few people know how to create a healthy spiritual living process because they have been taught that happiness is to be experienced in the physical reality, which is a product of living with a flawed thinking process. Perhaps, the most important precursor for creating a healthy spiritual living process is love. A fact of life is that "we don't live well without love", and we suffer without love. The world would not last a day without love. In its place are acts of violence, and efforts to gain control and power, are all created by one's unhealthy ego. Furthermore, if not all our problems, at least most of them, are directly related to issues of love, beginning with not loving yourself. If you ask people what love is, you will probably never get the same response twice because we live at a time when we don't know what is real or not real. Furthermore, we seem to get our definition of love from Hollywood, and it goes something like the following. Two people connect, the excitement accentuates, they get married, have a family, have children, grow old, and live happily ever after, and it all happens within 90 minutes. This is what we want to believe.

However, this is a long way from happiness and love. Yet, when one stops and thinks about this, one should not be surprised we do not know what love is because we don't have many role models to show us. However, we use the word love for almost everything we like. For instance, you may have heard someone say: I love my car, I love that song, I love that color, I love my pet, and so on. Then there is love for children, love of God, a love of humanity, love of money, and love for your significant other. How strange that we use the word love so often, but really don't know what it is. Furthermore, we really do not know how to create love, yet we crave it.

When it comes to intimate relationships, we are a huge failure because we don't know what love is, or how to love in an intimate relationship. However, we have learned how to fall in love with an image, which is based upon a fantasy around the image of what we want and think how a relationship should be. However, the relationship is not based on a foundation of strong character, equal respect, each willing to give and nurture the relationship, and effectively communicating when there are disagreements. Consequently, our character flaws are overlooked, but will surface at some point and lead to a downward spiral to a point in which the relationship is no longer an enriching experience. If character flaws are serious, then one has to consider whether or not to begin a serious relationship, or how long to stay in a bad relationship. These are very difficult decisions because we often see what we want to see and not what is, and splitting up is usually a painful experience, which makes for a difficult decision.

Several signs of serious character flaws include: jealousy, controlling behavior, mistreating of animals, and frequent episodes of rage, being manipulative, perfectionism, a hard to control temper, not allowing anyone to get close emotionally, and being extremely moody are the most common symptoms. These character flaws are symptoms of unresolved core emotional issues that create an imbalance within our inner sense of self, which lead to a flawed thinking process. Character flaws have a heavy influence on our flawed thinking process, especially our loving relationships. Unfortunately, we crave love and quite often people will do most anything to get love, or what they think is love. Much of acting out sexual behavior are efforts to get love, but this attention rarely leads to love. Therefore, there is a high rate of sexual transmitted disease because people confuse having sex, as love. Sexually acting out is really about efforts to get love, feeling self-validated, and about power and control. However, the reasons for most sexual encounters are symptoms of a flawed self-definition caused by unresolved emotional issues. Outside the context of love and intimacy, what we call love making is an empty physical act. Beside spreading disease, it also creates shame and an erosion of self.

Another concern about intimate relationships is about the individual who gives all of themselves to their partner. This is always a set up for an emotional train wreck because such an individual lacks healthy boundaries, which results in a loss of power, control, and the erosion of self. Consequently, one also becomes vulnerable to manipulation, and for all kinds of abuse. In addition, such an individual will enter a free fall when the relationship abruptly ends, and is vulnerable to a nervous breakdown, suicide, seeking revenge, or getting in rebound relationships, which is never a good thing.

A basic principle about love is that it begins with loving oneself. If I am unable to love myself, then I am unable to love another individual because I cannot give what I do not have. Therefore, your first task is to create a loving relationship with yourself, which implies having the discipline to create healthy boundaries that will function as a guide for your decision-making process. This also creates a process for nurturing yourself. This self-loving process also requires identifying your faults, character flaws, and having the discipline to change these into positive qualities, and or not allowing them to interfere with the relationship. Lacking this capability will give way to an uncontrolled impulsive decision-making process influenced by emotional needs, wants, and desires, which will create a dysfunctional relationship. Trying to love a dysfunctional individual is putting energy into foolishness because love is not possible. In the end, it is about desperation, rescuing behavior, not knowing what love is, believing the other person will make you happy, and the fear of being lonely.

Furthermore, love is choosing to commit to the relationship, which includes accepting the flaws of your partner, if they are not too serious, because we all have some issues. Yes, love is a choice! Think of a time when you may been on a date, and you conclude that you do not have any interest to see your date again. For some reason, you noticed his/her issues and realize there is not a loving future. In essence, you made a choice.

Love is also about growing consciously and spiritually together. Both individuals accomplish this putting effort to nurture the relationship and working through difficult times. Loving relationships are about giving up one's ego, treating the other as an equal, otherwise there will be a power struggle, which can lead to the demise of the relationship. Loving relationships are also about agreeing to disagree and yet, respecting the others opinion, when there is a difference in beliefs and opinions. Loving relationships must create a comfort zone, which will free both individuals to communicate without fear of some sort of backlash or punishment. Lastly, they are about trying your best to stay together during tough times and growing together because difficult times will change the dynamics of the relationship. Tough times require patience, safe communication, good coping skills, and time to allow feelings and emotions to be processed. The outcome will help the relationship grow stronger, which should be the goal. Once you commit to relationship, it is important to strengthen and enrich the relationship daily. This can also be accomplished by implementing daily rituals as: both make dinner together, taking a walk together, watch a movie together, etc. Such rituals stimulate communication, a sharing of feelings, and the message of caring for each other.

However, we should not forget to mention this thing called infatuation, which is extremely intense and is characterized by a total collapse of self and boundaries. People often get infatuation confused with love, which it is not. In this period, each other smothers the other and there is frequent sex. However, this eventually ends, and the sense of self and boundaries snap back in place. Then everyone looks at each other in a different light because the excitement is over, and often, character flaws then surface and change their perception of each other and the relationship. There are times when infatuation can lead to a healthy relationship, but everyone will have to recognize their issues, and want to work on their issues together when the infatuation is over. This is when the real relationship begins but is usually a difficult process because we must realize that we have issues that may get in the way. Usually, both partners don't even realize that they have issues. A big mistake is to believe that he or she will change down the road, which rarely happens. Without addressing our emotional issues, they will rise to the surface, inflict their damage, and often destroy the potential of a loving relationship.

Many people have the perception that emotional infatuation, or excitement is love and these feelings should never end. Unfortunately, it does end, and often one partner will usually conclude the relationship is over. For such an individual, this infatuation is a drug and a very addictive drug. Furthermore, when it is no longer present in the relationship, a partner splits and begins the search for this infatuation with a new partner. Consequently, it is very common for this individual to get involved with one partner after another, which leads to a lot of emotional misery. This is a quite common cycle for highly dysfunctional people, and they repeat the cycle of falling in and out of love numerous times. Love for them is not possible because they lack a healthy self-definition, lack boundaries, and function with a flawed thinking process, which makes them incapable of love because they can't give what they don't have. Plus, they are looking for someone else to make them happy, which is not possible.

In essence, a healthy loving relationship begins with both partners having a healthy self-definition. Such an individual will also have parameters. Parameters that allow each other to enrich the relationship experience, which does not happen by itself. This must be created by creating a framework that allows for this enrichment. Parameters as: both individuals are equal, each will contribute to basic duties and responsibilities for maintaining a proper and healthy household, both will have their own checking account and effectively manage their money, both will create time for emotional intimacy, both will implement healthy living practices, both will give each other space, both will give appropriate emotional time to the relationship, both will contribute to the responsibilities for child rearing, both will communicate in a healthy manner, etc. Such parameters will create a framework that create healthy boundaries that guide the relationship for both individuals. That is, both will often be on the same page, experience minimal stress and strain on the relationship, and be able to effectively manage difficult periods.

Creating an Effective Thinking Process

Hlthy Self +	Effective +	Effective Mindset +	Everyday Living =	Life Outcome
Definition	Emotional	(Options, Tech Skills)	(Psych Needs)	Good Decisions
(integrity)	System	(Rules & Guidelines)	(Goals, Vision)	
(dignity)		(Essential EI, Beliefs)		

Creating a Healthy You!

Creating a new you begins when one begins the process of creating a healthy self-definition. The first step is to examine the life you are living, and if you admit that it is beyond normal, and or an unhealthy living process, then your life is a dysfunctional life. In essence, you have been living a lie. Yes, a lie because the moment you looked into the mirror, saw what you wanted to see, which was not the dysfunctional life you are living, you told yourself a lie. From this point on, you had to keep lying to yourself and to others. Overtime, you created a large web of lies, which protected your troubled living process. This is called denial.

The next step begins with identifying all the people who mistreated you or created some type of serious harm to you. I am sure we all have a lengthy list of people who have caused harm to us. Every day when you get up, say something like: _____ the hell with you. This will help you mentally end the harm and misery these people have caused you, and help you take control of the misery they caused. You must also tell yourself to no longer feel guilty, or shame because of what people did to you. Shamed and guilt are often left over emotional lingering symptoms of being harmed mentally and emotionally, and one must eradicate these symptoms before one can move on. Keep in mind that you have a right to love yourself and like yourself. Therefore, beginning today, whatever happened in the past, will not have a negative effect on creating a healthy you. Another important exercise is to forgive yourself for all the times you did dumb things to others, and realize you were a jerk at one time. Doing these things will help you create a clean slate that is necessary for discovering and creating the real you.

Creating a healthy self-definition is not easy because defense mechanisms have been created through childhood that protected you from the toxic family environment. This helped your cause for self-preservation, but there are psychological scars from your toxic ordeal that created your flawed self-definition. This can make the discovery process difficult because these defense barriers are difficult to break down. For some individuals, especially people over 50, breaking down barriers is extremely difficult because time has hardened them to almost a point of no return. However, with help from a professional therapist, hopefully, one can participate in the emotional work to dissolve some of these defense barriers. Yes, it is painful, but through the act of processing our emotional core issues, you will be freed from your emotional bondage, which will allow you to begin to create harmony and a sense of wholeness within, and free the human spirit.

One of the main healing points is to come to grips with the dysfunction of your family beginning with your parents. Yes, they had their issues and did the best they could, but it was not' good enough, and you can tell them that in several ways. This realization must be experienced before one can really continue through the healing continuum. During the healing process, one can then begin to learn to create healthy boundaries, and how to nurture yourself. Then one can become the real person they were meant to become by creating a new journey. Usually, one will have to seek professional help to deal with their emotional issues, but for many, they will not go until there is a serious life changing event because life changing events create total confusion. It is this confusion that often motivates people to seek help.

Things we can do to enhance our self-definition
* Make good decisions.
* Don't do things to get noticed.
* Treat others with respect.
* Participate in good things in school and in your community.
* Talk to a counselor, if you are troubled by something.
* Don't let your friends make your decisions for you.
* Consider the consequences of your decisions.
* Identify situations that could lead to trouble and avoid them.
* Create positive goals and devise a strategy to accomplish them.
* Don't hang around with people who get in trouble.
* Do good things for you: exercise, eat healthy foods, and get a hobby.
* Create healthy coping habits.

The following is a list of the many benefits that come with a healthy self-definition
* Experience pride and self-confidence.
* Create a healthy vision.
* Attract healthy friends.
* Develop healthy values.
* Better able to manage stress.
* Become more effective in finding solutions to problems.
* Create a better thinking process.

*   Develop healthy boundaries.

You have a right to create the real you, which is the beginning of creating a new journey. I urge everyone not to believe that your dysfunction is caused by a genetic flaw because you will see yourself as a victim. This is a small victory, but an important victory because without this, one will lack the will to become healthy and create a healthy self-definition. From this event, one can make progress in creating an effective thinking process required for creating a healthy journey. Every day people get up, and through some life challenging event, come to the realization that the life they are living isn't the one they want. They realize that they are getting consumed by the madness of their troubled living process and need to change. This is what happens when denial is broken down, along with defense mechanisms. People then can create an effective thinking process that can help to simplify their living process. Also, learn to create significant meaning, purpose, and hope because their true sense of self begins to blossom. All are trying to feel better, to be more confident, experience more love, and to enjoy being the real you, as you create a new living process.

Creating an Effective Thinking Process

Hlthy Self	+	Effective	+	Effective Mindset	+	Everyday Living	=	Life Outcome
Definition		Emotional		(Options, Tech Skills)		(Psych Needs)		Good Decisions
(integrity)		System		(Rules & Guidelines)		(Goals, Vision)		
(dignity)				(Essential EI, Beliefs)				

Creating an Effective Emotional System

Emotional health is a state of positive psychological functioning. It includes an overall experience of wellness in what we think, feel, and do through with the highs and lows of life. (Healthy Place, 2021). An important task is learning how to effectively manage feelings and emotions, but this depends upon having an effective emotional system. We know that a flawed emotional system is about mismanaging painful feelings and emotions, often repressing them into our unconscious believing they are forever gone. The accumulation of repressed feelings becomes a toxic stew that churns away within, creates havoc with our thinking process, and our physiological processes. In addition, this also becomes toxic to the human spirit because we will make bad decisions that create more shame-based feelings. Any feelings and emotions that we repress will always come back to haunt us. Old feelings die hard, and still water runs deep, are two accurate statements that describe repressed feelings and emotions. Before one begins to create an effective emotional system, one must go back and dig up traumatic old feelings and emotions related to serious life events. This is a painful difficult cleansing process, but a necessary one, if one has the desire to break free from their emotional prison. Don't hesitate to seek a professional therapist to help with this process.

The challenge is not to let painful feelings and emotions lead to self-pity thinking that overwhelms you and define you. Then begin to engage in positive coping strategies like giving yourself a pep talk. Think about how things could be worse and realize there are millions of people who are suffering much worse than you are. Think about all the good things that are in your life and appreciate them. Think of all the wonderful things, yet to be experienced. You can also begin to develop a plan that includes doing things that are positive like: taking a walk every day, remember the good times, keep a diary, and meditate, have a conversation with yourself, and with the universe, are a few things you can do that will help ease your pain, and to efficiently manage your feelings. It is also a good practice to have a discussion with yourself about the event, and ask yourself: If you were to give advice to a dear friend who experienced a similar event, what advice would you give him or her? You would probably give some good advice, so listen to it. Constructive behavior will also positively affect your feelings and thinking, which helps one look on the bright side. This is a good thing because this results in a feeling of control that resonates from within. Doing positive things and listening to your own advice, your spirit and positive energy will grow stronger, and you will create more clarity of your situation and your future. Consequently, you will become an active participant in your healing process, which is imperative, if you want to create purpose, meaning, love, and hope.

One of the unique things about being a human is that we can step back and engage in self-examination regarding how our life is playing out. This may be painful because we must see ourselves for who we are, and this may not be a good picture. In doing so one must identify their faults, weaknesses, and character flaws that are causing a troubled living process, which is filled with painful feelings and emotions. This will help one to understand that their flawed emotional system is working and is interfering with their living process. The next time you are feeling down, create a constructive plan that consist of doing positive things that will have a positive impact on your approach to dealing with everyday difficulties and the larger picture for living. A loss of control is common when feelings and emotions take over our thinking, which often leads to doing something stupid and feeling sorry for yourself, which only makes life more difficult. Never make life more difficult is a good rule to live by! If you find yourself in an emotional hole, do not dig it deeper. Creating a process to effectively manage your feelings and emotions requires you to examine your beliefs that set the tone for how you manage feelings and emotions. The following beliefs can help create a new process for effectively managing your emotional system.

* **Believe you will get through the situation.**
* **Ask: What can I learn from this situation?**
* **Believe that life will be good again.**

In addition, it is important to understand that humans are designed to have feelings and emotions, and it is ok to experience them. They make us feel alive and help us enjoy the living experience. Not to have them would be like a computer and never feel anything. There are individuals who are severely flawed emotionally, and do not know what they feel and are totally numb. Some people are just out of touch with their situation because their flawed thinking process creates confusion and chaos and their flawed emotional system malfunctions. Consequently, overtime, the buildup of feelings and emotions, reach a boiling point and there is a trigger event that blows the lid off. Such an individual will then have an explosion, which seldom produces a good outcome. Once we admit and recognize our feelings, then identify specific feelings and ask: **Why am I feeling this way**? This will help to recognize and honor our feelings. This will help us to become responsible for our feelings, which can help prevent a blow up. The following questions can help process feelings and emotions in a healthy way.

* What feelings did I experience today?
* What things made me upset, angry, frustrated?
* What am I feeling at this moment?
* Why am I feeling this way?
* How long did these feelings last?
* How did I contribute in creating these feelings?
* How do I see myself when looking into the mirror?
* How long do I want to feel this way?

Once we have answered these questions follow-up with the following.

* What can I learn from these feelings?
* Talk to someone about your feelings: you will always feel better.
* Keep a journal that describe your feelings.
* Do something positive like take a walk and give yourself a pep talk.
* Always think positive about yourself.
* Never be embarrassed to feel.
* It is ok to cry because it is a healthy release.
* Talk to a counselor, they can help you, to help yourself.

Most people have difficulty managing feelings and emotions within the normal stressors of the everyday ups and downs because of living with a flawed emotional system. Managing them becomes ever more difficult when there is a life changing event because there is a significant loss and change in the daily living process. In that, feelings and emotions become extreme, and totally upset the living process. Consequently, the everyday living process becomes more difficult to function on a normal level because of the chaos and confusion that is coated with anger, which often dominates the thinking process. In addition, meaning, purpose, love, and hope are diminished.

Anger is always the enemy, which always prevents people from moving on and creating a new normal healthy living process. Anger takes life from us! Furthermore, we often take our anger out on those closest to us, which drives them away. This only isolates us, and then we have less support and love, and loneliness becomes our companion. Yes, life gets worse. Most of us will have at least one life changing event because that's life. However, the many people living with a flawed thinking process will usually have many significant life changing events. That is, they will make many bad decisions that will lead to life changing events. When our dysfunctional living process is extreme, the individual will always live on the edge of their next crisis, which often creates our next life changing event.

When life changing events happen, you do have the power to change your thinking and create positive ways to cope that will get you through the situation in a positive manner. This is not easy, but it is the best option. Begin each day by taking a deep breath, step back from the situation, and look at the big picture, and realize that this is only a moment in time, which will pass into time. Your goal is to make sure you come out as a new healthy person, which requires that you effectively manage the painful situation. Also, realize that everyone has a lot to live for including you, and the present misery will fade away and become a memory with time, when processing with an effective emotional system. This will help you from engaging in self-pity and to effectively manage past painful feelings and emotions. Furthermore, view the situation as a challenge, and as an opportunity to change and create a new you, a new life, and that is exciting. Without growth, one will often see themselves as a victim and become encapsulated with anger.

Life changing events are usually related to love, which is the greatest source of joy and happiness, and the source for our greatest pain. Love anything, and it will leave you before you leave it, or it may die before you, or you will die before it. Consequently, it hurts when we lose something to which we are emotionally attached. Furthermore, when that person is no longer a part of our life, we must get emotionally unattached, and redefine ourselves, which is often a very painful consuming process. This other person contributed to your meaning, purpose, and love, and we do not live well when these things are diminished, and or gone. Moving on to create a new normal is exceedingly difficult, if we do not get over the initial shock of the event, especially if one has a flawed thinking process.

The first step in processing feelings from life changing events is to recognize that painful events can and will happen because it is a part of the living process. Dreadful things do happen, and often unexpectedly, which makes life very difficult. It is important to believe that everything has a beginning and an end. Hopefully, this will be a philosophical core belief because it will help in making a transition to a new normal way of living because it will minimize the anger. Anger is amplified when one does not expect painful things to happen because we are blindsided and in shock because we are unprepared mentally and emotionally. Consequently, we must manage and control our anger, which is difficult and sometimes can turn to extreme depression and anger.

The second step is that the sooner one accepts the event, the quicker one can begin to process the emotions and feelings, which will move us out of anger. The third step is that life changing events change people permanently, that is, their consciousness will be changed, which will lead to a different outlook about life, and a different daily living process. Hopefully, this change will be a positive change because you can create a new healthy normal way of living. This will help create new purpose, meaning, hope, and love. This healing process becomes a spiritual change, but only happens if we have a thinking process that allows it to happen. A common mistake during this life changing event is to try and live life the way it was prior to the event. This is a product from not accepting the event, and from living in fear of what might come with change. This fear, along with denial, often prevents one from moving to closure and creating a new healthy normal. Such an individual becomes emotionally stuck in one place, which is usually anger, and the human spirit will suffocate. Life changes, and we must have an effective thinking process to accept, move to closure, and create new purpose, meaning, love and hope. Life changing events are the universe's way to move us along the spiritual journey.

A Life Changing Event
Several years ago, I was in a beautiful mountain town where summers are spectacular. An older couple arrived to spend the summer months in their summer getaway. A friend and I unloaded their moving van, and they were incredibly grateful for the help because unloading would have been an arduous task because of their age. That evening I came back to check on how things were going. We sat on the porch with a glass of wine, and he began to share a life changing event. Early in their marriage, they lost their only child in a car accident. Dad refuses to accept this event, and for the next eight years was consumed by depression, anger, and rage, and his life spiraled out of control.

After eight years of living in extreme anger, he was mentally, emotionally, and spiritually bankrupt, and reached a point of suicide. It was at this time; he made the choice of participating in professional therapy. The therapist, through a lot of challenging work, was able to change his consciousness, moved him to acceptance, and this set the tone for the healing process to take hold. He restored his relationship with his wife, and then began to create a new healthy normal living process, and was able to create new meaning, purpose, love, and hope, which became a new healthy journey.

His intense anger began because he refused to accept the event of losing his daughter. In his thinking, this was not supposed to happen, and it was not fair. The outcome from this thinking was anger and rage that consumed him because his flawed thinking process was unable to process the painful feelings from the event. Overtime, his flawed thinking took him to the verge of suicide, which was the only solution his thinking process could produce at that moment. The sooner we can accept a life changing event, we begin to honor our feelings, and begin to process them. What follows is closure and the process of creating a new healthy normal living process.

It is extremely important to effectively process our feelings and emotions, otherwise, they will create a deep dark emotional hole that sucks life from us and destroys the human spirit. Usually, the outcome is a sense of hopelessness, a loss of hope, developing a reliance on mood altering behaviors, relationships are damaged, and then we live in isolation controlled by anger. This is not the journey we want to experience.

Creating an Effective Thinking Process

Hlthy Self	+	Effective	+	Effective Mindset	+	Everyday Living	=	Life Outcome
Definition		Emotional		(Options, Tech Skills)		(Psych Needs)		Good Decisions
(integrity)		System		(Rules & Guidelines)		(Goals, Vision)		
(dignity)				(Essential EI, Beliefs)				

Creating an Effective Mindset

Our mindset is the control center that directs our thinking process, which leads to decision-making process according to our reality, which creates our everyday living experience. It must enable one to successfully navigate the challenges and challenging times that one will experience. The outcome of successfully navigating the twists and turns of living, is to turn our experiences into purpose, meaning, love and hope. Failure to do so is to become overwhelmed by our emotional misery, which only leads to a troubled living process caused by a flawed thinking process that will diminish our sense of hope.

Our mindset is comprised of a belief system that has been shaped by our experiences, especially childhood experiences, and by our family, friends, social media, and religious beliefs. The belief system of many people pertains to making money, being successful at moving up the ladder, just do it, live in the moment, and enjoy. Presently, most children are provided a very protective childhood, and are also provided an amazingly comfortable living process that modern technology has provided. Physical work is a thing of the past, however, children must develop a degree of discipline, if they want to experience any degree of success in life. However, many children have little or no discipline, furthermore, they want everything right now to experience all the fun they can get, and to keep up with their peers. This is their reference point that governs their decision-making. However, they never have what they want, and always want more because more will make them happy. That is today, they will not be happy unless they have the latest IPhone or laptop, etc., which have become the new addiction. This is their reality; however, this belief system will fail them because its focus ignores their sense of self, which will be diminished because they are unable to create healthy boundaries and fail to nurture themselves. They then become susceptible to herd mentality, which for most, is allowing others to define them. That is, everyone is doing it, so it must be ok.

A major task for living effectively is to examine our belief system and to fine tune it, which is something few people ever do. An effective mindset is like a GPS system that will take you to your desired destination. However, the software for most people is comprised of an outdated belief system that leads to bad decision-making, bad outcomes, and a troubled living process. A function of an effective mindset is to observe events, sort through the events, analyze the information, then make an accurate conclusion, which leads to an accurate reality, and then create an effective solution, if required. An effective mindset will efficiently conduct each of these tasks and result in making good decisions that help create purpose, meaning, hope, and love.

The following are benefits of an Effective Mindset
* Plan a course of action if required.
* Determine the important things.
* Create a positive attitude.
* Help to recognize and process feelings.
* Identify potential strategies to manage experiences.
* Determine the real from the unreal.

As a society, we are having great difficulty in making good decisions because of a flawed thinking process. Presently, many people are being swayed by the Trump propaganda train, and unfortunately, they see what they want to see. Sadly, they fail to see the real man and how he suffers from extreme narcissism. An effective thinking process will help manage our thinking and help one to function in relation to an accurate reality. The following are some benefits from living with an effective thinking process.

* Make decisions with logic and reason.
* Take more time to decide.
* Minimize the emotional fall out from painful events.
* Maintain healthy values and create healthy boundaries.
* Make decisions with the future in mind.

Creating an effective thinking process requires an examination of existing beliefs that were discussed in the previous chapter. Many beliefs for most people are passed down assumptions that have become expectations that create a false reality, and false hope. Our false reality becomes the leading cause of frustration, which is an unfulfilled expectation, and one must be careful about creating unreasonable expectations. An effective mindset will allow for the examination of events, which will help in creating an accurate reality, which will lead to making good decisions. Below are some beliefs that make up an effective mindset that is efficient in creating an accurate reality.

Beliefs for an Effective Mindset
* Feeling good is not happiness.
* Life is perfectly fair and anything can happen to anyone.
* Having social status is not that important.
* He/she is not responsible for your happiness.

* Bad things do happen and are a part of life.
* Money is nice, but it cannot buy happiness.
* Children are a joy, but raising them is a very big challenge.
* We might live a happily ever life, but only if we work hard at it.
* Happiness is not having a new house.
* Living together does not prevent divorce.
* We need a job/career, but it is not the most important thing in life.
* Pain and suffering are a part of life, but don't let them lead to anger.
* Life is easier when we no longer try to control the uncontrollable.
* Love requires a lot of hard work.
* Relationships are difficult, but can be effectively managed, if we work at them.
* I cannot change anyone.
* We can work things out, but only if we work at our issues/problems.
* We will grow apart, if we don't work at staying together.
* Children will get in the way, if we don't commit to them.
* We will not always look good, and we will get old.
* Life is difficult, but we don't have to make it more difficult.
* It is only important that I do my best.
* Loyalty may not be returned, but if I do my best, I will have my self-respect.
* You will reap what you sow.
* Things may look better on the other side of the fence, but your side is what is important.
* All my problems will follow me.
* I am responsible for my problems, and my living process.
* I am never a victim.

Accumulatively, these statements form a belief system that provides an accurate reality, which is the basis for the development of an effective thinking process. Now we have a chance to manage life events, make good decisions using logic and reason relating to our integrity, and life goals. Consequently, we are actively involved in creating a quality living process that has meaning, purpose, love, and hope.

Understanding Rules and Guidelines and Effective Thinking
The purpose of an effective thinking process is to create a good decision-making process. However, there are life events that can push us to the edge of doing something stupid, which is what you never should do. For instance, life changing events create a lot of suffering and anger, which is a common outcome. Furthermore, making decisions based on anger, will always create more suffering, shame, and guilt. The function of rules and guidelines is to help one to remain cool, calm, and collective during periods of intense painful life changing events. This is achieved by controlling painful thoughts and maintaining an effective thinking process.

Rules and Guidelines for Effective Thinking

* Blame yourself and not others for your problems.
* Never make big decisions when emotionally distressed.
* Believe in you and never doubt yourself.
* Live in the present, plan for the future, don't live in the past.
* Forget the bad things from the past: don't carry a grudge.
* Think of your future when making decisions.
* Identify and take care of the things that are in your control.
* Protect and nurture your integrity: never compromise it.
* Keep life special, it's all we have, and the clock is ticking.
* Never take things personally.
* Keep an open mind: don't resist change.
* Keep your composure, or you will always have to patch things up.
* Don't let "but" keep you from following your dreams.
* Think positive things about yourself.
* Realize that no human being is bigger than life.
* Try hard to keep your life balanced.

Summary

A major challenge is to make good decisions during the ebbs and flows of the everyday living process and life changing events. Creating an effective thinking process can help to successfully navigate the difficulties of living by making good decisions, while keeping an eye on our future.

Creating an Effective Thinking Process

Hlthy Self	+	Effective	+	Effective Mindset	+	Everyday Living	=	Life Outcome
Definition		Emotional		(Options, Tech Skills)		(Psych Needs)		Good Decisions
(integrity)		System		(Rules & Guidelines)		(Goals, Vision)		
(dignity)				(Essential EI, Beliefs)				

We all want fewer problems that produce stress, sleepless nights, conflict, and basically make living a miserable experience. Many problems are created by poor communication skills that leads to conflict. Instead of listening and thinking about what was said, many people react with an intense attacking tone of voice, and or get defensive, or say nothing, which is not always a good thing, if you want to solve a problem. We could significantly improve the living process, if we would improve our ability to effectively communicate by using technical skills that can help improve communication, prevent problems, and prevent a bad situation from getting worse.

* Communication Skills
* Skills to Resist Peer Pressure
* Skills for anger management

* Steps for effective decision-making

I am sure you have seen conflicts and have conflicted with another. These are often intense, and everyone involved will experience painful feelings because of the conflict. Sometimes, conflict can lead to a violence, which is never a good thing. **Right?**

Our challenge is to avoid, and or prevent this conflict from happening. If not, we can learn to minimize the conflict and not have it escalate to violence. Below are some tips that can help you improve your communication skills (Peterson, 1987).

1. **Show Mutual Respect**. The attitude of one or both partners may be more important than the sticking point. Have the attitude that you want to solve the problem together, which is more important than trying to win because it is better that you both win.

2. **Pinpoint the Real Issue**. Identify what it is you are arguing about. Clarify the issues involved and think about them from all angles before you begin to discuss them. This way your energy can be directed at the right place and gets away from name calling and finger pointing.

3. **Seek Areas of Agreement**. Most people begin by focusing on what they do not agree on. Identify areas of what you agree on, how you think alike, and how you can change your behavior. The idea is to find a solution to the issue and not destroy the relationship.

4. **Mutually Participate in Decisions**. After some discussion, work out a tentative agreement or solution to the problem. If you cannot agree, then postpone making any decision, and return to it later. Also, accept the fact that you may not agree with each other, and that is ok. Remember, you are not trying to control the other person, but to find a solution.

5. **Be Specific**. Whatever the problem is, identify the facts, be specific about what is bothering you, and express your feelings. Do not wander into other things that have happened at some other time.

6. **Focus on the Present and the Future**. Often when people are discussing something, they will bring up past events. This only derails the interaction process. Focus on the present and the future.

7. **Use "I" Messages**. Starting your sentencing with "I" demonstrates that you accept responsibility instead of blaming the other person. It also allows the other person to see how you view the problem. It is a very important process because it **clarifies** the issues.

8. **Don't Try and Figure out who's wrong and who's right**. Trying to win or not to lose only derails the interaction process and may lead to not finding a resolution. The goal is to cooperate with each other to find a solution and not to compete. **Don't have any regrets**.

9. **Say What You are Thinking and Feeling**. The other person is not a mind reader, and they do not know what you want, or how you feel. Gently, say what is on your mind. Don't leave and then wish you would have said this or that. **Be Truthful!**

10. **Set a Time Limit for Discussing Your Problems**. Sometimes you can talk forever and never solve anything. If talking does not lead to anything productive, then stop talking, set a time to come back, and continue the discussion. **Stay focused!**

11. **Speak calmly with a soft tone.** Often, when discussing touchy subjects, everyone often communicates with an elevated tone of voice, which usually creates a tense situation worse. As concerns and accusations are expressed, this tone becomes more elevated, which is never a good thing because this may lead to aggressive verbal abuse, and or violent behavior. Generally, both partners will emotionally move away from each other when aggression occurs and both will experience more emotional pain. Overtime, this adds more emotional damage to the relationship, and even destroys the relationship because there is a point of no return. Keep in mind that screaming and hollering never does anyone any good, in fact, it only causes more emotional damage. When you feel your anger raising, take a deep breath, remain calm, and speak with a soft tone. This will allow the both of you to discuss the issue at hand, instead of trying to intimidate the other individual. Furthermore, it shows that you are concerned about the feelings of the other individual and probably lead to a solution.

The goal is to solve the issue at hand and not let it escalate into an intense argument. Poor communication skills will only result in causing pain and distance between each other. Think of it as an emotional disconnect. Consequently, both partners involved will have scarred feelings and emotions, which can destroy the relationship. Effective communication will help solve problems and nurture the relationships, which is the goal of the interaction.

Skills to Resist Peer Pressure
Instead of making our own decisions, many people are pressured into deciding that they really do not want to do but give in to pressure. This is called peer pressure. You may have experienced this pressure being around your friends or peers. They use this technique to get you to do something that you really do not want to do. Consequently, many people often make poor decisions even when they know the decision is the wrong decision. A good thinking process means that you must be able to resist peer pressure and make decisions using logic and reason in regards as to what is right and wrong. The following discussion describes specific verbal statements one can use to resist peer pressure (Hammes & Duryea, 1985).

The first one is known as having **personal credit**. Remember that you are a smart individual, and you do not have to do anything for anybody, nor do you have to prove anything to anybody. These statements indicate that you like who you are, and that you do not have to do anything to be anyone's friend.

1. You mean I must do this to be your friend?
2. If I must do this to be your friend: then I do not want to be your friend.
3. I like you guys and want to be your friend, but not if you want me to do bad things.
4. No, you should not force me to do something that I really don't want to do.

The next one that can be used to resist peer pressure is to **delay the decision**. The situation may change if you can stall because it gives you more time to think about the situation and all the consequences before deciding.

Delaying the Decision
1. Do I have to decide right now?
2. Let me think about it for a while.
3. Maybe I will do it some other time.
4. Begin talking about something else.

Another verbal skill is **recruiting** a friend or an ally, when you are in a difficult situation. This is a response that can be used when others have teamed up against you and are pressuring you to do something you do not want to do. The intent is to try and recruit someone to side with you, and to help redirect the pressure.

Recruiting a Friend
1. Ask a friend: Do you agree with them?
2. Ask a friend: Do you think I should do it?
3. Ask a friend: Do you think they are right?
4. Ask a friend: Are you going to do it?
5. Ask a friend: What are the consequences?

These are verbal skills that can be used when your peers are trying to make you do something that could get you into trouble or be harmful to you. Remember, a real friend will never make you do things that are bad for you. **Make Good Decisions!**

Anger Management
Let's talk about anger. We often get angry when we do not get our way, when people make fun of us, when people make us do something we do not want to do, when we get used, and manipulated, abused, or when life throws us a life changing event. Anger is a response to an unfulfilled expectation and being able to manage powerful angry feelings is a must.

What is quite frightening is that sometimes anger quickly turns to violence. There are many people in jail or prison because their anger quickly turned to violence. There is another source of anger, which comes from a terrible childhood. This person has a deep reservoir of anger that influences their decision-making the wrong way, and every now and then, anger rises to the surface and causes serious problems. A therapist can help this person manage this anger, but only if they want to be helped.

Understand that anger is a part of life and is necessary for survival. For example, if you are attacked, and your life is threatened, your anger will increase your adrenalin and strength because your survival instincts will kick in gear. However, rarely will any of us have to rely on this for survival. The goal with anger is not to let it destroy relationships nor turn to violent behavior. Learning to effectively manage anger can prevent a lot of problems. Anger management skills can help manage these intense moments when anger could erupt. Below are some dos and don'ts for managing our anger.

Don'ts
* Don't let anger control your thinking.
* Don't let anger lead to physical violence.
* Don't let anger control your tone of voice and the words you use.
* Don't let the anger of others make you angry.
* Don't let anger control other emotions
* Don't let anger make your decisions.

Do's
* Use anger as a signal that there are problems that need to be addressed, see a counselor.
* Take a deep breath and think before you speak.
* Take action when necessary, but only after you have carefully thought through the situation.
* Express anger in moderation without losing control.
* The goal is to solve problems and not just to express feelings.
* State your anger clearly in ways others can understand because then they can respond appropriately to your concerns.
* Always consider your options when you feel you are losing control.
* Always consider the consequences of possible decisions.
* When you have the urge to become violent do something physical like, taking a walk, slow your breathing down, write your feelings on paper or talk to someone.
* Finally, let go of your anger once the problem is resolved.

We can learn to prevent anger and to minimize its place in our life. It doesn't have to control our thinking and consume us, but only if we learn to think differently.

Remember: Anger that is Not Managed Can Turn to Violence: Prevent This!

Using an Effective Decision-Making Process
Every day we make important decisions without ever giving much thought how we made these decisions. A challenge for us is to use certain steps before deciding, and then we can make a

good decision. Let us look at the five steps that outline a thinking process that can be used to make good decisions (Furby & Beyth-Marom, 1992).
1. Identify all possible options in the situation.
2. Identify all possible consequences to the situation.
3. Evaluate the desirability of the consequences for each option.
4. Determine the likelihood of the consequences.

Few people engage in any thoughtful thinking process when making decisions. Furthermore, hardly anyone uses step four because most decisions are reactionary because of the impulsive influence of raw feelings and emotions, which lead to a bad outcome. An effective thinking process will use logic and reason, which should lead to consequences in relation to healthy goals. This step will always help in making good decisions and less emotional distress. For example, using drugs and sex for mood altering are two behaviors that few people ever think about the implications, and both can lead to horrific results at many different levels. Using these steps in your thinking process can help anticipate problems, avoid risky situations, and experience less emotional misery.

An Effective Thinking Process

Hlthy Self	+	Effective	+	Effective Mindset	+	Everyday Living	=	Good
Definition		Emotional		(Options, Tech Skills)		(Psych Needs)		Decisions
(integrity)		System		(Rules & Guidelines)		(Goals, Vision)		
(dignity)				(Essential El, Beliefs)				

Essential Elements
Essential elements are attributes that help prevent emotional misery, make good decisions, and helps to develop and maintain a positive attitude about self and about life. The following describe the importance of essential elements that can make living a little easier.

A Sense of Humor
This is about having the ability to laugh at oneself especially when in a difficult situation. It is about diffusing and releasing anger, and bad feelings in a positive way. People who have a sense of humor will not have much of a temper, and as a result are less likely to react with anger and violence. It makes a lot more sense to laugh at ourselves and at the situation, instead of doing something stupid that only intensifies the situation.

Being Optimistic about the Future
Despite the craziness in the world, it has always been crazy, you can still be optimistic because you can create a wonderful life by making good decisions in relation to your passion. You can create the life you want with an effective thinking process and that is exciting. Believing you have control of your life and can be resilient, and to adjust to the challenges, is especially important in living an empowered life. Look to the future and create a healthy loving future.

Patience

It is very difficult to experience success in life without having patience. Patience allows one to remain cool, calm, and collective, as compared to having a short fuse and losing your temper, which never does anyone any good. It also helps one stay on course to reach your goals. Patience allows good things to materialize.

Empathy

This means you can feel or sense the feelings of the other person. Living with empathy is about realizing that we all suffer and are vulnerable when we suffer. Do not judge or criticize because everyone does the best they can with their pain, and you don't know how you will react when you experience similar pain. Empathy will help to understand the pain and suffering we all experience and to provide support to those in need. It connects us to others because we are all the same and belong to humanity. It also makes life a little easier.

Creativity

People with a flawed thinking process usually resort to doing things the same old way when they are faced with stressful situations. A flawed thinking process created the problem and cannot solve the problem(s). Be creative and learn to solve your problems by thinking about creative solutions. You can always look at your problems differently, which can lead to creative solutions.

Adaptability

A flawed thinking process keeps people from being able to adapt to life situations and to make successful transitions during life changing events. Challenging times are common and can be short lived, if one can adapt. It is like making lemonade when life gives you lemons. It is not easy, but adapting makes living possible again, which is the best option.

Self-Discipline

This is a form of self-love. It is about having restraint, putting up with some discomfort, delaying gratification, and working hard to accomplish a goal before rewarding oneself. Self-discipline is required for experiencing any success and in creating a healthy lifestyle.

These are important elements that will help keep one focused on their goals, keeping life's difficulties to a minimum, and to keep life moving forward in a positive way. They will also assist in making good decisions based upon logic and reason. They can also help prevent emotional suffering and redirect energy towards our future. In essence, essential elements are important in creating and maintaining a healthy journey.

Options and Effective Thinking
An Effective Thinking Process

Hlthy Self	+	Effective	+	Effective Mindset	+	Everyday Living	=	Good
Definition		Emotional		(Options, Tech Skills)		(Psych Needs)		Decisions
(integrity)		System		(Rules & Guidelines)		(Goals, Vision)		
(dignity)				(Essential EI, Beliefs)				

Options

Options are very important for the development of a healthy lifestyle. A flawed thinking process limit's one's ability to create and identify options that might be the solution to the problem. We all face difficult life situations, and the challenge is to find the right solution for the problem. For instance, an individual who finds themselves in a place in life where they do not want to be, believe they cannot get out of the situation, or change their life for the better, is without options. In severe instances, they might believe they are stuck, feel imprisoned, have lost their sense of power, had an over loaded emotional system, and often believed they are a victim. Such a person often believe they do not have options, which results in a loss of power and control that will lead to a loss of hope that life will get better. The result, without some form of treatment, is the suffocation of the human spirit, which will manifest as a deep depression, and or a nervous breakdown. In this confused mental state of mind, their thinking process failed them, they lose sight of the important things in life, and lose their sense of self. This is a very scary moment because they begin to lose their reason to live.

My mother and aunt experienced a nervous breakdown caused by a flawed thinking process. Growing up, I wondered why they had a nervous breakdown and knew that I did not want one. I also said to myself, someday, I want to discover the cause of a nervous breakdown. To find the cause I had to dig up the family history, which produced some remarkably interesting stories. It was clear that my mother and aunt made several bad decisions that lead to a life they didn't want, and the emotional distress was overwhelming. Both were unable to create purpose, and meaning, and therefore, they loss their hope that life would get better. The result was a loss of power and control that led to them giving up because they were overcome by guilt, shame, and depression. Their flawed thinking process failed them and giving up was the only option they had. This created a sense of helplessness and hopelessness, which led to a nervous breakdown. My mother did recover, but my aunt never did. However, my mother had a second nervous breakdown in her later years and spent her last few years in total misery. Her flawed thinking process won again. Keep in mind that any traumatic experience in a family, or severe family dysfunction will impact all family members, and they then become the next generation that lives with a flawed thinking process and a troubled living process.

An effective thinking process can prevent a nervous breakdown because it considers multiple options, and provides a sense of hope, and freedom. It also maintains one's sense of power and nurtures the human spirit. Be creative and keep living. An effective thinking process is creative because it allows an individual to create and consider multiple options to life situations. This maintains one's sense of power, control, and protects and nurtures our sense of self and the human spirit.

Process of Everyday Living

An Effective Thinking Process

Hlthy Self	+	Effective	+	Effective Mindset	+	Everyday Living	=	Good
Definition		Emotional		(Options, Tech Skills)		(Psych Needs)		Decisions
(integrity)		System		(Rules & Guidelines)		(Goals, Vision)		
(dignity)				(Essential EI, Beliefs)				

An important component for making good decisions is understanding the psychological dynamics that occur during the everyday living process. Understanding the dynamics can help one to effectively prevent, manage and minimize stress, confusion, and misery. Psychological needs play a role in understanding the dynamics of how stress and confusion that occur in the everyday living process. In essence, there is a psychological underpinning to everything we do. That is, psychological factors motivate one to respond with a behavior. For example, have you ever found yourself driving behind a large truck, and you cannot see? Of course, when you got a chance, you passed the truck, and it was the psychological factors of freedom and the sense of control/power that motivated you to pass. Goals also play a critical part for creating an effective thinking process because they will create a positive vision, and a strategy that will lead to a better future that includes purpose, meaning, love, and hope.

* Satisfy psychological needs
* Have short- and long-term goals
* Creating a positive vision

Each day we face a fast paced, demanding, competitive, and non-forgiving grind. It is like running through a maze, hoping to find a way out, but never do, and each day we lose a little bit of ourselves. Yet, we get up and try again, only to experience the same day we had the day before, like the movie Ground Hog Day. For many CEO's, individuals in administration, and people in sales, are often told to do better, and work harder to get better results. Whatever their efforts are, or were, it is never enough. Well, something must give when you continue to give more of yourself, and usually one then has less time and energy for themselves, and for their loving relationships. Eventually, many lose their sense of self and reach a breaking point, which can lead to unwise decision making with bad life outcomes. Our life experiences occur within the following areas:

* Our family, work, relatives, and friends.
* Relationships/dating, school, and children.
* Community, money management, and social life.
* Private life, environmental issues, and job.
* Aging, country, planet.

These areas are where life happens. It is where the expected and the unexpected happens. This is where we are supposed to create purpose, meaning, love, and hope, but we are failing at this task. A contributing factor for experiencing failure in the above areas is the inability to satisfy psychological needs, and we suffer when these are not adequately satisfied. They are directly related to the experience of our general well-being. William Glasser (1984) describes these psychological needs.

Psychological Needs

Another reason we experience a lot of suffering is because we are unable to satisfy psychological needs. Most people do not even know that these exist, yet most of our efforts are our best attempt to fulfill some need. Unfortunately, most people have the desire to feel good and use destructive behaviors to make them feel good. The cause is a troubled living process that fails to satisfy these psychological needs. Think of the behaviors you have used to feel good. We will always feel better and happier when we have fulfilled our psychological needs in a responsible manner. We will experience emotional frustration when we are unable to get these needs met in a positive way. Some symptoms experienced include anger, depression, and anxiety, which often motivate people to look for a quick mood alteration.

An important aspect related to our experience of health, happiness, and general well-being is dependent in our ability to adequately satisfy our psychological needs. William Glasser (1984) describes these needs.

1. Belonging (Love)

Our need to belong, to love others, and to be the recipient of love from others, is as important, as having food and shelter. This need occupies a large part of our lives, and we experience a great deal of emotional misery when we do not adequately satisfy this need. Belonging is believing you are a valued member of the family, the community, and connecting in a loving way with others. Participating in events or being an active member by serving on special committees, is also an investment in your community and in humanity. These activities create a feeling of belonging, a sense of connecting with others, and love for humanity.

2. Power

Our greatest frustrations occur when we attempt to control others because we discover that no one can really control anyone. People without power are likely to suffer from a poor self-definition and will become susceptible to manipulation and exploitation by others.

Consequently, their self-definition will be compromised, and they will be full of anger and depression. We often compete against each other for power instead of negotiating it, and having respect for others, and accepting each other as equal are very important for having power and maintaining it. The power we need to think about is having the ability to control and manage our emotions, feelings, and thinking, and in making good decisions. This implies creating healthy values and boundaries, which allows us to effectively manage our living process. Power is a need for survival, fulfillment, satisfaction, and happiness. **Do not give it away, and don't misuse it.**

3. Freedom
Can you think about life without freedom? What kind of life would you experience without it? The ability to make good decisions, to experience happiness, and to fulfill your dreams is dependent upon freedom. We lose our freedom when we allow someone else to control us and to make decisions for us. We lose freedom when we live in a troubled living process because our needs, wants, and desires control us, and take our freedom of choice. Many not only give their power away, but also give away their freedom, and then create a situation of dependency. Living without freedom will result in the experience of anger, fear, self-doubt, and hatred. Without freedom, life becomes a life never lived. Personal freedom implies that we love ourselves, accept full responsibility for our lives, and make good decisions. **Do not lose your freedom.**

4. Fun
An important element in life is to have fun. Fun for many is watching TV. Then there are many who believe that having fun is doing dreadful things like using drugs or other destructive behaviors. This is not fun! It is pleasure seeking behavior, and symptomatic of an inner disturbance, and a flawed thinking process. Fun is having good friends, loved ones, and doing things that are not harmful to them or to you. Fun can also be experienced through activities like enjoying a few moments of peace and quiet, a walk-in nature, or watching a sunset. Fun is also working with others, accomplishing a goal, and doing anything that is positive. Fun is being healthy and engaging in things that nurture life in a healthy manner. **Learn to have fun!**

Remember, we experience painful feelings when we are unable to satisfy our psychological needs. Then we feel dissatisfied and just feel miserable. Over time, we often chose a destructive coping behavior to make bad feelings go away. Now that we know what these needs are, we can learn how to fulfill them in a responsible way. We will then feel good about ourselves and experience more moments of feeling good. In addition, you are beginning to create a healthy journey.

Goals are Dreams Waiting to Become Reality

Life Goals

Take a few moments and think about your future. That is right, your future! The future will come, and it does not matter if you are happy or not. It just happens. Let us develop a plan that creates a future of purpose, meaning, hope, love, and less suffering. Without goals, your life will wander like a ship, with nowhere to go. It is like taking a trip, but you do not have a map to show you the direction to get to your destination. Without positive goals your life will lack direction, and purpose, meaning, and hope, will be diminished. The result is a meaningless day-to-day living process with no joy. Life then often becomes a boring, unfulfilled, and miserable experience without positive goals. Positive goals provide the incentive to achieve, they help us channel our energy and give us hope. Satisfaction, pride, and self-confidence are experienced when we achieve our goals. These are all positive experiences. Positive goals are dreams waiting to become reality. Positive goals can enrich your life experience.

Please realize that often long-term goals are often dependent upon you having and achieving short term goals. For example, let us say you want a job that will allow you to travel the world, but if you don't graduate from high school, you will most likely never leave home. However, goals that only serve your immediate satisfaction will not provide happiness and fulfillment. Think of famous movie stars. Most have had the goal of acquiring fame and fortune and have successfully fulfilled these goals. However, many have addictions and many other destructive behaviors that are destroying their lives. So, what is missing?

Many people often have goals that are only about the experience of success related to making money, acquisition of things, and getting more things. These goals ignore the important things in life, like creating healthy relationships and loving relationships. These relationships are what is most important in one's living process, and they should be top priority in creating a healthy journey. We must have some goals that address love, compassion, and kindness because this is what life is about.

Goals should help you to enrich the experience of purpose, love, meaning, and hope.

Summary

The experience of everyday living is difficult because of our flawed thinking process that leads to bad decision-making and a troubled living experience. Please realize that anyone who lives this way struggles with purpose, meaning, hope, and love, and living begins to become an empty experience.

Final Thoughts

Below are all the components that we have discussed that can create an effective thinking process. A process that will lead to a healthy state of mental, emotional, and spiritual health. In essence, our well-being.

An Effective Thinking Process

Hlthy Self	+	Effective	+	Effective Mindset	+	Everyday Living	=	Good
Definition		Emotional		(Options, Tech Skills)		(Psych Needs)		Decisions
(integrity)		System		(Rules & Guidelines)		(Goals, Vision)		
(dignity)				(Essential EI, Beliefs)				

Take a few moments and think about the life experiences that you don't want.
* No one wants to spend any part of their life in jail or prison.
* No one wants to get into a bad relationship.
* No one wants to be hurt by someone else, or to hurt someone else.
* No one wants other's to use them or exploit them.
* No one wants to give up their total freedom to someone else.
* No one wants to have their friends make bad decisions for them.
* No one wants to live a life of extreme loneliness.
* No one wants to be dependent upon others for their happiness.
* No one wants to be poor.
* On one wants to experience a life that is full of misery.
* No one wants to become an addict.
* No one wants to become mentally or emotionally disabled.
* No one wants to die young.

Life is difficult and we don't have to make it more difficult, by living with a flawed thinking process. A thinking process that leads to making bad decisions that result in bad outcomes. Thus, a troubled life. The good news is that no one is a victim! You can learn to create and maintain a healthy state of mental and emotional health by learning an effective thinking process. Consequently, you can learn to make good decisions guided by healthy values and goals. In addition, you can experience: 1) peace of mind, 2) experience harmony, 3) find your passion, 4) coping well with the highs and lows, 5) having love in your living experience, 6) create and enjoy a simple life, 7) being centered and balanced, 8) able to nurture yourself, 9) being adaptable, and 10) being resilient. A healthy mental and emotional state of mind is essential for creating meaning, purpose, love, and hope, during all stages of our life. The spiritual life is waiting for you, just take the first step and begin the process of learning an effective thinking process, which creates a spiritual journey. With time, this thinking process leads to **illumination**!

Benefits Include
* Having a good thinking process.
* Not letting friends make your decisions for you.
* Identifying consequences of your decisions.
* Not to manipulate others for your benefit.

* Developing a plan for the future.
* Not making decisions for instant gratification.
* Getting help when you feel troubled.
* Learning from your mistakes.
* Not to blame others for your problems.
* Creating healthy boundaries.
* Learning how to nurture yourself.
* Preventing stress.
* Successfully managing your stress.
* Finding creative solutions for your problems.
* Protecting your integrity.
* Having positive coping behaviors.
* Never repress your feelings.
* Creating a healthy vision.
* Creating healthy relationships.

You Can Create a Great You and a Good Life!

References

Amazing Grace, Wikipedia

Drugfree.org 2021

Friel, J. & Friel, L. (1988) Adult Children: The secrets of dysfunctional families. Health Communications, Inc.

Furby, L, & Beyth-Marom, R. (1992) Risk taking in adolescence. A decision-making perspective. Developmental Review, 12, 1-44

Glasser, W. (1984) Control theory. Harper & Row.

Hammes, M. & Duryea, E. (1985) Teaching verbal and cognitive resistance skills to a sixth-grade population. J. of Human Behavior and Learning. Vol. 2, No. 1. Pp. 19-25.

Healthy Place, 2021.

Hemfelt, R., Minirth, F., & Meier, P. (1989) Love is a choice. Thomas Nelson Publications.

Mental Health.gov. May 28, 2020

Nakken, C. (1996) The addictive personality, Hazelden Foundation.

National Health Statistics, 2018.

Peterson, S. (1987) How to defuse fights before they fester, USA Today, April 17.

Shakespeare, Leaves of Gold, Coslett Publishing Co. 1963

Shapeinmind.com (2020) https://shapeinmind.com Carl Jung: Striving for wholeness and the unconscious mind.

Statistics (ncadv.org)